THE

USES OF WATER

—— IN ——

Health and Disease.

A PRACTICAL TREATISE ON THE BATH,
ITS HISTORY AND USES.

By J. H. KELLOGG, M. D.

PUBLISHED AT
THE OFFICE OF THE HEALTH REFORMER,
BATTLE CREEK, MICH.

1876.

PRINTED IN
THE UNITED STATES OF AMERICA

Facsimile Reproduction

Copyright © 2001 TEACH Services, Inc.
ISBN 978-1-57258-085-5
Library of Congress Catalog Card No. 97-60504

Published by
TEACH Services, Inc.
www.TEACHServices.com

PREFACE.

Since the announcement of the alleged discovery of Priessnitz, about fifty years ago, there has been no scarcity of books upon "Hydropathy," "Water-Cure," and kindred topics. With rare exceptions, these works have been, in reality, little better than advertising mediums for some individual or institution. As might be expected in works prepared for such purposes, they have contained numerous and flagrant exaggerations of the effects of water as a remedial agent, often representing it as a specific for certain maladies and a sure preventive of others. These extravagant accounts, together with various absurd teachings relating to methods of application, have rendered just the popular verdict indicated by the fact that the dingy shelves of nearly every second-hand book store in New York and Philadelphia, as well as other large cities, are laden with these musty old volumes which rest beneath the accumulated dust of years.

The objects of this work may be briefly summarized as follows :—

1. To present a careful and candid account of the nature of water and its physiological effects.

2. To explain the effects of water when used as a remedy for disease, and to demonstrate its value as a remedial agent.

3. To show that the employment of water in the treatment of disease has been practiced by the most eminent physicians of all ages, and is not a modern discovery.

4. To expose those absurd and erroneous practices which have brought the use of water as a remedy into disrepute, and have thus deterred scientific physicians from adopting it.

5. To provide a convenient manual of the various methods of applying water.

The reader will observe that water is not presented as a panacea. Its use is not advocated as a specialty. It is only recommended as one of the many potent agencies which may be successfully employed in the treatment of the numerous ills to which humanity is subject—a remedy which has been abused by quacks and tyros and disgraced by fanatics, but which still urges a just claim to the attention and consideration of all candid persons.

J. H. K.

Battle Creek, Mich., Sept., 1876.

CONTENTS.

USES OF WATER

IN HEALTH AND DISEASE.

PHYSICAL PROPERTIES.

WATER is one of the most abundant elements in nature. As rivers, lakes, seas, and oceans, it covers three-fourths of the earth's surface. It even enters largely into the formation of the solid rocks. The clearest and purest air contains it in large quantities as an invisible gas; while in clouds, fogs, and mists, it appears in the form of minute drops.

Water also forms a very considerable part of all vegetable productions, and constitutes about *three-fourths* of the human body, as well as other animal tissues. The blood and the brain are each about four-fifths water, while the fluid secretions and excretions contain more than nine-tenths of their weight of this limpid fluid.

Chemical Composition.—The chemist designates water as hydrogen oxide, and represents it by the chemical formula, H_2O, which signifies that it is composed of the two gases, hydrogen and oxygen, in the proportion of two volumes of the former to one of the latter. Both of these gases are colorless, transparent, tasteless, and odorless. Hydrogen is the lightest gas known; oxygen is the great supporter of combustion and animal life and heat. Water is produced by the burning, or oxidation, of hydrogen, a process attended with very little light, but most intense heat. The two gases are explosive when mixed.

Physical Properties.—Water exists in three states; viz., as a solid, in the form of ice; as a liquid, its most common form; and as a vapor, in the form of steam. When in the last condition, the gaseous, it is invisible. That to which the term steam is very commonly applied, is not steam, but water in a state of fine division, or mist.

Below 32° F., pure water exists in the form of ice. Between 32° and 212°, it is a liquid. At 212°, it is converted into vapor. Water also slowly evaporates at all temperatures below 212°, being absorbed and held in solution by the air.

Water possesses the greatest specific heat of any substance. By specific heat is meant the actual amount of heat required to elevate its temperature a given number of degrees. For example, it requires ten times as much heat to raise a pound of water 1° in temperature as to elevate a pound of copper 1° in temperature. To raise the temperature of a pound of lead 1°, requires only one-thirtieth as much heat as to produce the same effect upon a pound of water. Water absorbs more heat by elevation of temperature than any other substance. In passing from the solid to the liquid state, it absorbs a vast amount of heat without any elevation of temperature. The same thing occurs in the conversion of water into steam or vapor by evaporation. In the evaporation of one pound of water, as much heat is absorbed, or rendered latent, as would suffice to raise nearly a thousand pounds of water one degree in temperature. This heat is abstracted from surrounding objects; and, hence, evaporation is one of the most powerful means of producing cold. The effect is the same, no matter what the temperature at which evaporation occurs.

Water is not the best conductor of heat, but it conducts much more readily than air, and readily communicates its heat to bodies with which it comes in contact, also abstracting heat when of a lower temperature, when changing from a solid to a liquid state, or from the liquid to the gaseous condition.

One of the most useful properties of water is its power to dissolve numerous substances, its solvent properties being nearly universal. To this property it owes its value as a cleansing agent.

Pure Water.—Absolutely pure water is not found in nature. Rain water is the nearest approach to it; but even this gathers impurities of various sorts as it falls through the air, and often becomes very unwholesome by the absorption of foul gases and the collection of dust in this way. For any use connected with the human body, the purest water is always preferable to any other. Filtered rain water and distilled water are the purest forms of water attainable.

Hard Water.—Water is said to be hard when it will not produce a good lather with soap, but forms curds instead. Hardness is due to the presence of earthy salts in the water; salts of lime—chalk and gypsum—are the most common. Ten grains per gallon of any of these salts is sufficient to render water hard and unfit for use, though some waters furnished to cities for general use contain from 70 to 160 grains per gallon of solid matter. Hard water is unfit for cleansing purposes because its mineral ingredients form insoluble compounds with fatty substances. When mixed with soap, the lime or other mineral takes the place of the soda or potash in the soap, and forms an insoluble curd, instead of a lather.

Mineral Water.—Water containing in solution salts of iron, magnesia, or other metallic elements, as well as sulphur, arsenic, iodine, or any compound of these or other elements which are capable of imparting a nauseous or saline taste, an unpleasant odor, or medicinal properties, has been much employed for the cure of all sorts of chronic ailments. Such waters are totally unfit for general use for drinking or cooking purposes, and certainly possess no particular advantages as cleansing agents. Whether they are useful as medicines is a medical question which we do not purpose to consider here; but one would naturally suppose that water which is unfit to cleanse the outside of the body could not be of very great utility as an internal application.

Magnetic Water.—Within the last few years, the scientific world has been startled with the alleged discovery of "magnetic wells" and "magnetic springs" in various parts of the country. The claim has been made and stoutly defended by interested parties that the water furnished from these sources is magnetic in character, and possesses wonderful healing virtues on that account. The truth in the matter, when viewed in the light of science, seems to be that the water of these much-lauded wells is no more magnetic than any other water; the magnetic phenomena are all explicable by well-known laws of physics, without attaching to the water any magnetic properties. A close examination shows that the iron pipe through which the water passes is the only magnetic object. The supposition that the pipe derives its magnetism from the water is both unnecessary and illogical. In the first place, any iron pipe or rod placed vertical in the ground

—or, better, placed parallel to the earth's axis—will spontaneously become magnetic. The production of magnetism is greatly favored by the friction of flowing water, and by jarring, as beating with a hammer. In the second place, the water possesses no magnetism to impart. In view of these facts, the conclusion is inevitable that so-called magnetic water has no existence except in the minds of certain persons whose credulity greatly exceeds their scientific knowledge.

"Magnetic" wells and springs are ingenious humbugs. Thousands of people are duped by them. Hundreds are benefited by getting well washed, and by enjoying recreation and pleasant social surroundings. The curative effects are attributed to the imaginary magnetism, while other more tangible agents are the real means of cure.

HYGIENIC RELATIONS OF WATER,

In order to be able to appreciate the value of water as a means of preserving health, it is necessary to understand something of the structure and functions of those portions of the body to which it is directly applied; viz., the skin, externally, and the mucous membrane, in the interior of the body.

STRUCTURE OF THE SKIN,

The skin is composed of two principal layers; a thin outer layer, called the epidermis, cuticle, or scarf skin, and a deeper structure, the true skin, or dermis. We will describe the latter first.

The True Skin.—This structure covers the entire surface of the body. It varies in thickness according to its location, being thickest upon the soles of the feet, the palms of the hands, the back, and the outer portions of the thighs. Its basis is a dense network of elastic fibers, among which are intricately mingled minute blood-vessels, nerve fibers, and lymphatic or absorbent vessels. These are most numerous near the upper surface, and are arranged in loops upon little elevations called papillæ. In the palms of the

hands and upon the soles of the feet these papillæ
are disposed in rows with so much regularity as
to give to those parts a minutely furrowed appearance.

The skin also contains little sacs, or follicles, in
which the hairs originate. In its deeper portions
are found two kinds of glands; sebaceous glands
for the secretion of sebaceous or fatty matter to
lubricate the skin, and the perspiratory or sweat
glands, the latter of which will receive a more
definite description shortly.

The Cuticle, or Epidermis.—At the upper portion of the true skin, new cells are being constantly formed, which become old in a short time and
are pressed outward by the formation beneath
them of other new cells. The old cells become
shriveled and flattened as they grow older, and
by a continuation of the process described, numerous layers of cells are formed upon the surface of the true skin, the lowest of which is
composed of newly formed cells, while the up-
permost one is made up of dessicated cells having
more the appearance of horny scales than of cells.
These several layers constitute the epidermis, or
outer skin. It is totally devoid of sensibility, and
has no blood-vessels. It is, in fact, dead, and is
useful only as a protection to living parts beneath.

Scattered among the cells of the epidermis are
colored cells, which give to the skin its proper
color. In the Caucasian race, these cells are few;

in the negro, they are abundant; while in the albino, they are wholly absent.

The Sweat Glands.—A close examination of the little ridges found upon the palms of the hands, by the aid of a small magnifying glass, will reveal what appear to be fine transverse lines crossing the ridges at short intervals. A still closer inspection shows that the apparent lines are really minute openings, guarded by delicate valves. These are the mouths of the perspiratory ducts, which convey to the surface the product of the sweat glands. The gland itself is merely a coiled tube, already described as situated deep down in the true skin, and is surrounded with a net-work of blood-vessels. The duct is simply a continuation of the same tube upward through the cuticle to the surface. It passes out upon the surface of the skin obliquely, thus leaving a small portion of the cuticle overlapping its orifice, forming a sort of valve.

The number of these delicate glands is enormous. It has been carefully estimated to be about 2,300,000 in a single individual. The length of each is about one-fifteenth of an inch, making their aggregate length about two and one-half miles.

The Mucous Membranes.—All cavities in the body which communicate with the surface by openings are lined with a membrane which is called mucous, from the character of its secretion. The mucous membranes are continuous with the skin at the natural openings of the body, and very closely resemble it in structure, being formed of several layers, like the skin, and having a superficial portion made up of layers formed by the deeper tissues. Mucous membrane forms the lining of the air-passages and lungs, of the whole alimentary canal, and of the urinal and genital organs. Its extent in the lungs alone has been estimated by scientists at 1400 square feet, or more than seventeen times the whole extent of the skin.

Functions of the Skin.—The skin performs a number of very important offices for the body. Perhaps the most important is that of excretion. Each of its millions of sweat glands is actively and constantly engaged in separating from the blood impurities which would destroy life if retained. These foul products are poured out through a corresponding number of minute sewers, and deposited upon the surface of the body to the amount of several ounces each day, or several pounds, if the whole perspiration be included in the estimate, as is commonly done.

The skin is also an organ of respiration; it absorbs oxygen, and exhales carbonic acid gas, with other poisonous gases. The amount of respiratory labor performed by the skin is about one-sixtieth of that done by the lungs. In some of the lower animals, the whole work of respiration is performed by the skin. In the common frog, the respiratory action of the skin and of the lungs is about equal.

Another important office of the cutaneous tissue is absorption. The absorption of oxygen has been already referred to; but it absorbs liquids as well as gases, and to a much greater extent. By immersion in a warm bath for some time, the weight of the body may be very considerably increased. Dr. Watson, an English physician of note, reports the case of a boy whose weight increased nine pounds in twenty-four hours solely by cutaneous absorption of moisture from the air. This extraordinary action was occasioned by disease. Seamen, when deprived of fresh water, quench their thirst by wetting their clothing with sea-water, the aqueous portion of which is absorbed by the skin. The lymphatic vessels are believed to be the principal agents in absorption.

Another remarkable function of the skin is the regulation of temperature. By its density and non-conducting property it prevents the escape of necessary heat to a considerable degree. But when the amount of heat generated in the body becomes excessive, either from abnormal vital activities, or by exposure to external heat, the skin relieves the suffering tissues by favoring the escape of heat. This desirable end is attained through the evaporation of the moisture poured out upon the surface by the perspiratory glands. It has been estimated that the evaporation of water from the cutaneous surface and the mucous membrane of the lungs occasions the loss each minute of sufficient heat to raise a pint of water 100° F. in temperature. This is certainly a powerful cooling process.

Lastly, we mention as a further function of the skin, and one which is not the least in importance, its utility as a sensitive surface. It is a well-established physiological fact that the mind is only a reflection of impressions received from without, or at least that its character is largely determined by the nature of the impressions made upon its organs of sensibility. The skin is the organ of touch, and the various modifications of tactile sensibility. It is the most extensive organ of sensibility in the body, and is very closely connected with all the great nerve centers, so that it is perhaps the most efficient means through which to affect the general nervous system. Its intimate sympathy with internal organs is shown in a great number of diseases in which this organ evidently suffers on account of disability of some other one.

Functions of the Mucous Membranes.—The functions of the mucous membranes are strictly analagous to those of the skin. Like the latter organ, a mucous membrane excretes and absorbs. It eliminates foul matters, and absorbs useful substances in a fluid state.

The importance of the functions of the skin is

shown by the fact that a person quickly dies when its action is interrupted. A coat of varnish or caoutchouc, applied over the whole skin, will kill a man almost as quickly as a fatal dose of strychnia. In experiments upon animals, horses, dogs, and other animals have been killed by obstructing the action of the skin by some similar means. A little boy was once killed by covering him with gold leaf to make him represent an angel at a great celebration.

The offensive odor of the perspiration, and the characteristic smell of the sweat-soiled underclothing of a tobacco user, are facts which well attest the value of the cutaneous functions in removing impurities from the body.

We are now prepared to consider, understandingly,—

The Hygienic Value of Water.—If we except pure air, it may safely be said that no other element in nature sustains so important relations to the living system as does pure water. An individual will live much longer on water alone, than if deprived of drink. Water constitutes a large proportion of all our food, varying, in grains and vegetables, from fifteen to more than ninety per cent. If the water thus contained in solid food were wholly removed, an individual would doubtless be enabled to subsist longer on water only than on solid food so treated. Though water undergoes no change in the body, and hence takes no part in the development of force, it is absolutely essential to the performance of the vital functions, being necessary to enable the various organs to perform their offices in the maintenance of the vital activities.

The circulatory system is especially dependent upon this element. Water is the menstruum which floats the blood corpuscles and the varied nutritive and excrementitious elements which form the blood. By its aid, the nutrient particles destined to enter into the structure of the body are conveyed to the most minute and remote fiber of the intricate human mechanism where repair or growth is demanded. No other element in nature is so well suited to this exact purpose as water. It is so limpid and mobile that it can circulate through the most delicate capillaries without friction, and can even find its way, by osmosis, into parts inaccessible by openings.

Thirst.—Water is continually passing away from the body. The dry air entering the lungs by respiration absorbs it from the moist surface of the pulmonary membranes. A large portion is lost by evaporation from the skin, upon which it is poured out by millions of little sewers, the perspiratory ducts, for the purpose of washing away impurities from the system. The kidneys remove a considerable quantity, with poisonous excrementitious elements in solution. Through still other channels water is removed, aggregating, in all, the amount of five pints in twenty-four hours in the average individual. This loss must be made good, in order to preserve the requisite fluidity of the blood; and nature expresses the demand for water by thirst.

Some people rarely drink liquid of any kind. Others consume several pints in a day. The nature of an individual's occupation will in a measure determine the amount of drink required. Stokers, glass-blowers, and others whose vocation necessitates profuse perspiration, require more water than others. It will be noticed, moreover, that the character of the diet has much to do with the demand for drink. Those who subsist mostly upon fruits and grains, and other vegetable productions, avoiding the use of stimulating and irritating condiments, require little or no addition to the juices contained in their food. Those who pursue an opposite course in dietetics, using largely animal food, salt, pepper, spices, and other condiments, and perhaps taking a little wine or something stronger for their stomach's sake, are under the necessity of taking considerable quantities of fluid in addition to that provided by their food.

Water is the only substance which will quench thirst. Beverages which contain other substances are useful as drinks just in proportion to the amount of water which they contain, and are unwholesome just in proportion as the added elements are injurious.

Regulation of Temperature.—The evaporation of water from the surface of the human body is one of the most admirable adaptations of means to ends exhibited in animal life. All of the vital activities in constant operation in the body occasion the production of heat. Sometimes the amount of heat is greater than is needed, and so great as would destroy the vitality of certain tissues if it were not speedily conducted away. By evaporation of water from the skin, this is accomplished. When external heat is great, perspiration is more active than when it is less, and thus the temperature of the body is maintained at about 100° F. under all circumstances. By this wonderful provision of nature, man is enabled to exist under the great extremes of heat and cold presented in the frigid regions at the poles and the torrid climate of the equator. By the aid of clothing, human beings have survived a continued temperature of 60° to 100° below zero; and, by the protective influence of evaporation, an average of 100° above zero has been endured in tropical climes. For short periods, so great a degree of heat as 350° F., or even 600° has been borne with impunity in exceptional instances. In these cases the extreme heat which would otherwise reduce the body to a cinder in a few moments is rapidly conducted away by evaporation without occasioning any damage.

Depuration.—Every thought, every movement, the most delicate vital action, occasions the destruction of a portion of the living tissues, which is thus converted into dead matter, and becomes poisonous. Many kinds of poisonous substances are produced within the body in this way. Some of them are very deadly, and must be hurried out of the system with great rapidity, as *urea* and *cholesterine*. Here the marvelous utility of water is again displayed. It dissolves these poisons wherever it comes in contact with them, and then as it is brought by the current of the circulation to the proper organs—the kidneys, liver, skin, lungs, and other emunctories—it is expelled from the body, still holding in solution the animal poisons which are so rapidly fatal if retained.

Cleanliness.—The skin is one of the most important depurating organs of the whole body. From each of its millions of pores constantly flows a stream laden with the poisonous products of disintegration. As the water evaporates, it leaves behind these non-volatile poisons, which are deposited as a thin film over the whole surface of the skin. As each day passes, the process continues, and the film thickens. If the skin is moderately active, three or four days suffice to form a layer which may be compared to a thin coating of varnish or sizing. The accumulation continues to increase, unless removed, and soon undergoes further processes of decomposition. It putrefies, rots, in fact, and develops an odor characteristic and quite too familiar, though anything but pleasant, being at once foul, fetid, putrid, pungent, uncleanly, and unpardonable.

But the offense to the nose is not the extent of the evil. The unclean accumulation chokes the mouths of the million little sewers which should be engaged in eliminating these poisons, and thus obstructs their work. Being retained in contact with the skin, some portions are reabsorbed, together with the results of advancing decay, thus repoisoning the system, and necessitating their elimination a second time.

Here water serves a most useful end if properly applied. It is unexcelled as a detergent, and by frequent application to the skin will keep it wholly free from the foul matters described. The necessity for frequent ablutions is well shown by the fact that nearly two pounds of a poison-laden solution, the perspiration, is daily spread upon the surface of the body. It is not an uncommon occurrence to meet with people who have never taken a general bath in their lives. Imagine, if possible, the condition of a man's skin, at the age of seventy or eighty years, which has never once felt the cleansing effects of a thorough bath!

One of the most serious effects of this accumulation of filth is the clogging of the perspiratory ducts. Their valve-like orifices become obstructed very easily, and depuration is then impossible. It is not wonderful that so many people have torpid skins. The remedy is obvious, and always available.

How to Make the Skin Healthy.—A man who has a perfectly healthy skin is nearly certain to be healthy in other respects. In no way can the health of the skin be preserved but by frequent bathing. A daily or tri-weekly bath, accompanied by friction, will keep the skin clean, supple, and vigorous. There is no reason why the whole surface of the body should not be washed as well as the face and hands. The addition of a little soap is necessary to remove the oily secretion deposited upon the skin.

A lady of fashion, in enumerating the means for preserving beauty, says: "Cleanliness, my last recipe (and which is applicable to all ages), is of most powerful efficacy. It maintains the limbs in their pliancy, the skin in its softness, the complexion in its luster, the eyes in their brightness, the teeth in their purity, and the constitution in its fairest vigor. To promote cleanliness, I can recommend nothing preferable to bathing. The frequent use of tepid baths is not more grateful to the sense than it is salutary to the health and to beauty. . . . . . By such means, the women of the East render their skins softer than that of the tenderest babe in this climate." " I strongly recommend to every lady to make a bath as indispensable an article in her house as a looking-glass."

When the foul matters which ought to be eliminated by the skin and quickly removed from the body are allowed to remain unremoved, the skin becomes clogged and inactive, soon loses its natural luster and color, becoming dead, dark, and unattractive. When bathing is so much neglected, it is no marvel that paints, powders, lotions, and cosmetics of all sorts, are in such great demand. A daily bath, at the proper temperature, is the most agreeable and efficient of all cosmetics.

Bathing Protects against Colds.—It is an erroneous notion that bathing renders a person more liable to "take cold, by opening the pores." Colds are produced by disturbance of the circulation, and not by opening or closing the pores of the skin. Frequent bathing increases the activity of the circulation in the skin, so that a person is far less subject to chilliness and to taking cold. An individual who takes a daily bath has almost perfect immunity from colds, and is little susceptible to changes of temperature. Colds are sometimes taken after bathing, but this results from some neglect of the proper precautions necessary to prevent such an occurrence, which are carefully stated elsewhere in this work.

Aristocratic Vermin.—Doubtless, not a few of those very refined and fastidious people who spend many hours in the application of all sorts of lotions and other compounds to the face and hands, for the purpose of beautifying those portions of the skin exposed to view—while neglecting as persistently those parts of the skin protected from observation—would be very much surprised to learn the true condition of the unwashed portions of their cutaneous covering. They instinctively shrink with disgust from the sight of a vermin-covered beggar, in whose cuticle burrows the *acarus scabiei* (itch-mite), while troops of larger insects are racing through his tangled locks and nibbling at his scaly scalp. It is quite possible that many a fair "unwashed" would faint with fright if apprized of the fact that her own precious covering is the home of whole herds of horrid looking parasites which so nearly resemble the itch-mite as to be at least very near relatives, perhaps half-brothers or cousins. The name of this inhabitant of skins unwashed is as formidable as the aspect of the creature, though it does not require a microscope to display its proportions, as does the latter; scientists call it *demodex folliculorum*.

The *demodex* makes himself at home in the sebaceous follicles, where he dwells with his family. Here the female lays her eggs and rears her numerous progeny, undisturbed by the frictions of any flesh-brush, and only suffering a very transient deluge at very long intervals, if such a casualty ever happens. In studying the structure of these little parasites, we have found several tenants occupying a single follicle, pursuing their domestic operations quite unmolested by any external disturbance.

The *demodex* has been transplanted from the human subject to the dog; and it is found that the new colony thrives very remarkably, and soon produces a disease apparently identical with that known as "mange."

We have not space to describe in detail these savage little brutes, with their eight legs, armed with sharp claws, bristling heads, sharp lancets for puncturing and burrowing into the skin, and their powerful suckers for drawing the blood of their victims. We only care to impress upon the mind of the reader the fact that neglect of bathing and friction of the skin is sure to encourage the presence of millions of these parasites, and that the only remedy is scrupulous cleanliness of the whole person. Like their relatives, the itch-mite, they do not thrive under hydropathic treatment, and are very averse to soap and water. The best way to get rid of them is to drown them out. They do not produce the irritation which characterizes the presence of the itch insect, so that this evidence of their presence is wanting. But they are sure to be present in a torpid, unhealthy, unwashed skin, no matter how delicate or fastidious its possessor.

Prevention of Disease.—Neglecting to keep the skin active and vigorous by frequent ablutions is one of the most prolific causes of nearly all varieties of skin diseases, which are too often aggravated by gross dietetic habits. The relation between the cutaneous function and that of the kidneys is so intimate that neglect of the kind mentioned, resulting as it must in obstruction of function, is a very common cause of most dangerous disorders of the renal organs. Inactivity of the skin is also very commonly associated with dyspepsia, with rheumatism, gout, hysteria, and other nervous derangements. It is also a not uncommon cause of bronchial and pulmonary affections. It is quite evident, then, that the proper and most efficient means of preventing these diseases is to maintain the functional vigor of the skin by the proper application of water.

The value of water as a prophylactic, or preventive, of disease, was recognized by the ancients, and the bath was employed by them to an extent which has never been equaled in modern times. The great Hebrew lawgiver, Moses, enjoined upon his followers the most scrupulous cleanliness, making bathing a part of their religious duties. His example was followed by the ingenious founder of Mohammedanism, who required his disciples to bathe before each of their five daily prayers. Among the Greeks, and especially the temperate Spartans, the bath was regarded as one of the most essential means of securing physical health. Daily ablutions were practiced by them, every person participating in the bath, from the new-born babe to the oldest inhabitant. The Romans cultivated bathing to a remarkable extent, making it a luxury rather than the dreaded penance which many moderns seem to regard it.

Modern Neglect of the Bath.—The most celebrated physicians, from Hippocrates down to Galen, Celsus, Boerhaave, and a host of more modern physicians, have agreed in eulogizing the bath as an invaluable means for preserving the health. Notwithstanding this fact, it seems that as civilization and enlightenment have advanced, the importance of the bath has been increasingly disregarded. The magnificent public baths of the Romans were neglected as that empire declined, until they were finally destroyed. Michelet, a historian of some note, tells us that for a thousand years during the Dark Ages the bath was unknown in Europe. This fact alone is in his opinion sufficient to account for the terrible plagues and pestilences of that period. A modern writer declares that in Spain the religious instincts of the people have become so perverted that it is considered sacrilege for a woman to bathe more than once in her life, which is upon the eve of her marriage. In more enlightened countries, it is to be hoped that the condition of the feminine cuticle is not quite so bad as this;

but another writer, an Englishman, asserts that a large proportion of his countrymen "never submitted themselves to an entire personal ablution in their lives, and many an octogenarian has sunk into his grave with the accumulated dirt of eighty years upon his skin." American customs in this respect are not much better than the English; but it is gratifying to know that a very perceptible improvement is becoming evident in both countries. Our intercourse with Oriental nations and barbarians has taught us wholesome lessons in the care of the person. There is scarcely a savage tribe to be found in the deepest jungles of tropical Africa the members of which do not pay more attention to the preservation of a clean and healthy skin than the average American or Englishman.

Bathing a Natural Instinct.—All nature attests the importance of the bath. The rain is a natural shower bath in which all vegetation participates, and gains refreshment. Its invigorating influence is seen in the brighter appearance, more erect bearing, and fresher colors, of all plants after a gentle rain. The flowers manifest their gratitude by exhaling in greater abundance their fragrant odors. Dumb animals do not neglect their morning bath. Who has not seen the robin skimming along the surface of the lake or stream, dipping its wings in the cool waters, and laving its plumage with the crystal drops which its flapping pinions send glittering into the air? No school boy who has ever seen the elephant drink will forget how the huge beast improved the opportunity to treat himself to a shower bath, and perhaps the spectators as well, for he is very generous in his use of water.

If man's instincts were not rendered obtuse by the perverted habits of civilization, he would value the bath as highly and employ it as freely as his more humble fellow-creatures, whose instinctive impulses have remained more true to nature, because they have not possessed that degree of intelligence which would make it possible for them to become so grossly perverted as have the members of the human race. Man goes astray from nature not because he is deficient in instinct, but because he stifles the promptings of his better nature for the purpose of gratifying his propensities.

PHYSIOLOGICAL EFFECTS.

SOME of the relations of water to the living system have been considered in the preceding section. In the present connection we shall consider chiefly those effects resulting from the application of water to the human body in various ways which give to it its value as a remedial agent, though its therapeutical applications will be deferred to succeeding sections.

The effects of water upon the human system are the results of the operation of its physical properties in conjunction with the vital forces. As with all other agents, its effects may be either local, or general, according to the mode of application. Different effects are also produced according as the administration is internal or external. Many other modifying circumstances, as age, sex, and physical condition, affect the results in a greater or lesser degree.

Water affects the system through three different means; viz:—

1. As a diluent;

2. By its solvent properties;

3. By modifying the general or local temperature of the body.

1. Water as a Diluent.—Water is received into the system by absorption, either through a mucous membrane, or through the skin. It usually enters through the medium of the stomach and intestinal canal. When received into the blood, it of course increases its volume, and produces an increased fullness of the circulatory vessels, which are never distended to their fullest extent, and hence allow room for change in the volume of their contents. The blood is necessarily rendered more fluid, and if previously in any degree viscid, its circulation is quickened by its dilution.

2. The Effects of the Solvent Properties of Water.—With the exception of air, water is the most transient of all the elements received into the body. It is eliminated by the skin, the lungs, the kidneys, and the intestines. By its solvent action, it dissolves the various poisonous products of the disintegration of the tissues. The volume of the blood being increased, more water comes in contact with the debris contained in any part, and, in consequence, the same undesirable products are more perfectly removed. The increased amount of excrementitious matter in solution is brought in contact with the various depurating organs, producing, notably, the following results :—

a. *An increase of the urinary excretion.* It is an important fact that this increase does not consist in the addition of water merely, or dilution, but that there is also an increased amount of *urea,* the chief excrementitious principle removed from the blood by the kidneys.

b. *An increase in the cutaneous excretion.*
Water drinking is one of the most efficient means
of producing copious perspiration, which, as with
the urinary excretion, is not a mere elimination
of water, but is a real depurating process.

c. *Increased action of the intestinal mucous
membrane.* Elimination from the mucous membrane of the intestinal track, which is an important organ of excretion, is also increased by drinking freely of pure water. The result of this increased action is not only to remove from the
blood some of its foulest constituents, but to render more fluid the contents of the intestines, and
thus tend to obviate that almost universal accompaniment of sedentary habits, constipation.

The removal of clogging matters from the system in this manner allows greater freedom of
vital action, so that the activities of the body are
quickened, and both waste and repair, disintegration and assimilation, are accelerated.

The use of water thus hastens all the vital
processes by increasing the change of tissue.
This result is of course chiefly obtained by employing it as a drink. The experiments of Liebig fully confirm this view. He expressly men-
tions the free use of water as one of the means
of accelerating vital change. Prof. John B. Bid-
dle, M. D., in his "Materia Medica," states that "it
promotes both the metamorphosis and construction of tissue," from which fact he attributes to
it valuable curative properties, as an alterative,

when the removal of a morbid taint is desired, as in certain venereal diseases.

3. Effects resulting from the Modification of Temperature.—Perhaps the most important, certainly the most common, effects of water upon the living organism are those which result from its modifications of the temperature of the body in its various modes of application. These effects vary greatly according to the temperature, and the duration of the application. General and local applications also differ in their results.

It should be remarked that all of the effects of water are really the results of the vital resistance of the system in its attempts to remove abnormal or unusual conditions, or to accommodate itself to new circumstances.

Baths are divided into six classes, according to their temperature, as follows :—

1. Cold, ... 33° to 60° F.
2. Cool, ... 60° " 70°
3. Temperate, ... 70° " 85°
4. Tepid, ... 85° " 92°
5. Warm, ... 92° " 98°
6. Hot, ... 98° " 112°

For the sake of simplicity, we will consider the effects of water applications under three heads ; viz., cold, warm, and hot.

The Cold Bath.—Under this head we will consider applications of all temperatures below 85° F. Cold or cool water, applied to any portion of the body, causes instant contraction of the small arteries of the part, through its influence upon the sympathetic or vasomotor system of nerves. So long as the application of the unusual temperature is continued, the vascular contraction is maintained, and the part seems nearly bloodless. If the cold is below 33° F., and is long continued, destruction of the tissues, by freezing, will result.

If a moderately cool or cold temperature is maintained for some time, the blood-vessels of the part are more or less permanently contracted, and the blood supply thus lessened. If, on the other hand, the application is very brief, the contraction of the vessels is only momentary, and is followed by a proportionate degree of relaxation, and a corresponding increase in the supply of blood to the part.

A very cold bath applied to any considerable portion of the body, and continued more than a very brief time, produces headache, dullness, sometimes nausea and vomiting, loss of sensibility, and other unpleasant and painful symptoms.

It is thus seen that the effects of cold are quite different—exactly opposite, in fact—as the application is a prolonged, or a brief one. The long application produces effects in some degree permanently sedative, while the brief application is followed by a momentary condition which may be termed shock, and which is usually followed very quickly by a reaction analogous to stimulation when produced in any other manner.

Effect of Cold upon the Pulse.—The experiments of Drs. Currie, Bell, and others, show conclusively that the cold bath has the uniform effect of diminishing the frequency of the heart's action from ten to twenty beats in a minute below the usual standard. Upon the first application of cold, there is a slight increase in the rate of pulsation; but this soon subsides, and is succeeded by a marked diminution. The ultimate effect is the same, whether the application is made at its maximum degree of severity or not; but if the application is first warm, being gradually reduced in temperature, the result is reached without the occurrence of the unpleasant shock, or feeling of chilliness, which attends the sudden application of cold, especially in persons of delicate nervous sensibilities. The amount and after duration of the diminished rate of pulsation depends upon the temperature and duration of the bath. In health, it does not commonly extend beyond a few hours at most.

Effect of Cold upon Temperature.—It was also shown by the same experimenters that the temperature of the body is reduced proportionately with the action of the heart. The natural temperature, as shown by a thermometer placed in the axilla, is 98° F. During and after a cold bath, the thermometer applied to the same part, indicates from one-half a degree to five or six, or even more, degrees, diminution of temperature. In some cases the temperature continues to fall after the bath. The real temperature is lessened even though the skin may glow, and may seem to possess increased warmth. Cold and heat are, within certain limits, wholly relative terms to the nerves of sensibility. What is warm at one time may be cold at another, though the temperature remains the same. The same temperature may be warm to one hand and cool to the other. Temperature can only be *accurately* determined by the thermometer.

Rationale of Effects of the Cold Bath.—The manner in which the cold bath produces the sedative effects noted, is apparently simple. When applied locally, to a single organ or part, it diminishes the circulation in the part by occasioning contraction of the muscular coats of the *arterioles*, or small arteries. Their caliber being thus lessened, they of course allow the passage of less blood, and the circulation in the part is diminished. There are, then, three causes for the decrease of heat; viz.,—

1. A portion of the heat of any part is brought to it by the blood; the supply of blood being lessened, the heat is diminished;

2. Heat is produced by vital or chemical changes which occur in the capillaries or their immediate vicinity. These depend chiefly upon the supply of oxgen, which, again, is largely regulated by the blood supply; and it being lessened

with the blood, the amount of heat *produced* is diminished.

3. The water in contact with the part, being of a lower temperature, abstracts heat from it as it would from any other body of a higher temperature than itself.

When the application of cold water is more general, being made to the whole body, or to a considerable portion of it, the same effects are produced on a larger scale. A large proportion of the small arteries of the body, being brought under the influence of cold, are made to contract, thus directly lessening the circulation, and so diminishing, also, the production of heat. Through the sympathetic system, the same effect produced upon the small arteries is produced also upon the heart, lessening the rapidity of its contractions. Again, it has been satisfactorily shown that the action of the heart is largely controlled by the action of the small arteries; so that we have abundant explanation of the decrease in the rate of pulsation. Finally, we have a cold fluid in contact with a large portion of the body, abstracting heat by conduction, as well as lessening its production.

Thus we see that water, when applied at a proper temperature, is one of the most powerful means of depressing the vital activities of the body, diminishing circulation and animal heat as will no other agent. The several modes for applying it are considered in another portion of this work.

The Hot Bath.—We shall include under this head applications of a temperature above 98° F., the mean temperature of the body. As with the cold bath, the effects differ greatly according as the application is brief or prolonged. Local and general applications also differ in their effects.

A brief local application causes an increase in the circulation of a part which very closely resembles, perhaps is identical with, active congestion. The small arteries are distended, and the vital activities and heat of the part are increased. The several effects seem to be little different from those resulting from the application of a mild sinapism. The action of the vital instincts is defensive in both cases.

When applied to special organs, special effects are produced. For instance, a hot fomentation applied to the head for a few minutes will usually produce drowsiness by diversion of a portion of the blood supply of the brain to the skull and scalp. Prolonged applications produce a more or less permanent relaxation of the blood-vessels, and consequent congestion.

A hot bath applied to the whole body, or a large portion of it, produces an acceleration of the pulse and an increase of animal heat proportionate to the temperature of the bath. A bath at 106° to 108° F. will increase the pulse from the normal standard to one hundred or one hundred and twenty beats in a minute, in a short time. A bath four or five degrees hotter has been known to increase the pulse to more than one hundred and fifty beats in a minute.

When a hot bath is prolonged, the face becomes flushed, and the whole skin very red; the head aches; sight is sometimes dimmed; ringing in the ears, faintness, a stinging pain in the skin, and intense desire to urinate are symptoms which are often present. Copious perspiration and intense congestion of the skin are constant effects. The cutaneous congestion, from relaxation of the blood-vessels, is apt to continue to exist after the bath, if it is greatly prolonged, to the serious injury of the subject.

The effects of the **vapor-bath** are essentially the same as those described, though a somewhat higher degree of heat is tolerated without injury. In the hot-air bath, a still higher heat is borne with impunity.

Rationale of Effects of the Hot Bath. — It scarcely need be repeated that all of the effects noticed, as well as those of all other baths, are chiefly the results of modifications of vital action occasioned by the agent employed. The application of heat to the body occasions relaxation of the muscular coats of the small arteries, and increased action of those vessels. No doubt this is for the purpose of bringing moisture to the surface to protect the tissues against the unnatural heat. As is the case with cold baths, the causes which modify the heat are three; viz.,—

1. The increased quantity of blood circulating through the part brings to it an increased amount of heat;

2. Increased vital and chemical action increases the production of heat;

3. The body absorbs heat from the surrounding medium as any other colder object would do.

In the general application of hot water or vapor, effects similar to its local effects are produced upon the whole surface of the body, involving, also, to a considerable extent, the deeper structures. The pulse is accelerated because the small arteries are distended and more active, creating a demand for a greater quantity of blood, requiring an increase in the heart's action. It is also quite probable that the action of the heart is somewhat quickened as the result of the influence of heat upon the pneumogastric nerve which controls it.

The cerebral symptoms, faintness, etc., which occur when heat is applied in excess, are the result of the diversion of so large a proportion of the blood into the superficial vessels. A prolonged hot foot bath or leg bath will often produce faintness.

There are few agents which will so rapidly produce such powerfully excitant and stimulant

effects as the hot bath. The painful and undesirable results occasioned by its incautious use
are evidences of its power.

The Warm Bath.—In this connection we apply the term warm to baths of a temperature
between 85° and 98° F., though baths of a temperature between 85° and 92° would be more accurately termed tepid, which term is applied to
baths of that temperature elsewhere than in this
immediate connection.

The warm bath never exceeds the temperature
of the body, and is usually below it. Its effect
is uniformly to diminish the frequency of the
pulse and of respiration, and to decrease animal
heat. Its effects are the same as those of the
cool or cold bath, in this respect, but they differ
in several other particulars. Unlike the cold
bath, the warm bath is not accompanied by an
unpleasant shock, or chill, and, hence, is not followed by reaction. It promotes the action of the
skin in a very marked degree, increasing both
perspiration and absorption. When continued
for an hour or two, the weight is appreciably
increased by the absorption of water. Its general effects are very mild and soothing, often in-
clining the patient to sleep.

This bath seems to produce its effects not so
much by exciting the vital energies to abnormal
action or resistance, as by supplying the most
favorable conditions for the performance of the

natural and usual functions. This is doubtless on account of its close approximation to the temperature of the body. In this respect, if this supposition be true, it differs from baths of a temperature either much above or greatly below the normal temperature of the body.

The warm vapor bath produces effects quite analagous to those of the warm water bath. Its effect upon the processes of perspiration and absorption is a little more marked, even with the same degree of temperature. The results differ somewhat, according as the whole body is enveloped, so that the warm vapor is taken into the lungs, or the head excluded. A more equable effect is produced by including the whole body in the bath, and no harm can result if the temperature is not raised above that of the body, as it should not be, in the *warm* bath.

Sympathetic Effects.—There is scarcely room for doubt that many of the effects of the various kinds of water applications are wholly of a sympathetic character. All portions of the body are intimately associated together by a system of nerves called the sympathetic system, from their peculiar function. Certain portions, as the skin and mucous membrane, are particularly related. The large number of sensitive nerves which connect the skin with the brain, bring it in peculiarly close relations to that organ, and give additional potency to any agent applied to so extensive

a surface. The well-known fact that burns of
the skin are often the occasion of fatal ulceration
of the mucous membrane of the intestines sufficiently attests the intimate relation between
these two tissues; while the effects upon the
skin of mental emotions, as of shame and of fear,
are conclusive evidence of the peculiar closeness
of relation between the cerebral and cutaneous
organs. The condition of the mind has much to
do with the effect of a bath.

Modes of Administration.—There are numerous modes of administering baths of all temperatures, each of which produces some modification
of the general effect of the given temperature.
For example, such baths as the douche, the spray,
and the shower bath, are much more cooling in
their effects than a full bath at the same temperature; since, in the latter case, nearly the whole
body would be submerged in a medium of equable
temperature, while in the case of the spray, etc.,
the body would be additionally cooled by the
rapid evaporation taking place upon its surface.
Many other peculiar effects are obtained by particular modes of administration, which will be described in their proper place.

HISTORY OF WATER CURE.

THE utility of water as an agent in the treatment of disease is not a modern discovery, as the pretensions of some aspirants for notoriety have led many to believe. A very cursory glance at the history of various ancient nations furnishes sufficient evidence that the use of the bath as a curative agent was of very remote origin. The works of the oldest medical authors contain numerous references to the bath, recommendations of its use in cases of disease, and testimonials of its good effects when properly employed. As this is a matter of some interest to many of those who employ and advocate the use of water as a remedial agent, as well as to those who are investigating its merits, we shall devote a little space to a sketch of the use and estimation of the bath by various nations and tribes—civilized and barbarous—and regular and irregular physicians, from the remote ages of antiquity down to modern times. For several of the facts presented we are indebted to a valuable work by Dr. Bell, long out of print and now somewhat rare.

The Bath in Egypt.—That bathing was practiced to a considerable extent by the Egyptians at a very early period, is evinced by both sacred

and profane history. It was through obedience
to this custom that Moses was discovered among
the rushes by Pharaoh's daughter as she went
down to the river side to bathe. Pictures discovered in ancient Egyptian tombs represent persons
preparing for the bath. We have no expression
of the estimate which was placed upon the bath
as a remedial agent; but it is hardly possible to
believe that an agent held in such high esteem
as a preventive of disease should not be valued
as a useful remedy.

Bathing among the Jews.—The code of laws
prepared by Moses, under divine instruction, for
the government of the Hebrew nation after its de-
parture from Egypt, made bathing a prominent
feature. The connection of the bath with the
treatment of leprosy would naturally lead to the
conclusion that it was employed for its curative
effects.

Persian Baths.—The ancient Persians held the
bath in such high esteem that they erected magnificent public structures devoted to bathing.
The baths of Darius are spoken of as especially
remarkable.

The Bath among the Greeks.—The cold bath
was employed among the Greeks. Lycurgus, the
famous Spartan legislator, prescribed its daily
use for all his subjects, not excepting the tenderest infants. In later times, the warm bath was

introduced, and stately buildings were erected for the accommodation of bathers.

The learned Greek, Hippocrates, the father of medical literature, and a very acute observer of disease and the effects of various agents upon the body, highly recommended the use of water in many diseases, describing with great care the proper mode of administering a simple bath. He laid great stress upon the careful and skillful use of the bath, asserting that, when improperly applied, it, "instead of doing good, may rather prove injurious." His directions for the employment of the bath were very discreet. He very wisely remarks that those patients whose symptoms are such as would be benefited by bathing should be bathed, even though some of the requisite conveniences may be wanting; while those whose symptoms do not indicate the need of this remedy, should not employ it, though all the necessary appliances are at hand. He made great use of water as a beverage in treating disease.

Roman Baths.—The Romans excelled all other nations in the sumptuousness of their bathing arrangements. Their public baths were among their greatest works of architecture, and were supplied with every convenience for increasing the utility and luxury of the bath. Kings and emperors vied with each other in perfecting and enlarging these sanitary institutions. Accommodations were provided, in some cases, for nearly 20,000 bathers employing the baths simultaneously; and at one time the number of public baths in Rome was nearly one thousand. Even Nero, whose name has come down to us covered with infamy, has the credit of doing at least one good act in erecting a magnificent public bath, though even the detergent effects of such an act can hardly cleanse his character of the many foul blots by which it is rendered odious.

Celsus and Galen, two noted Latin physicians, extolled the bath as an invaluable remedy, almost two thousand years ago. The latter pronounced the bath to be one of the essential features of a system of perfect cure which he termed *apotheraphia*, exercise and friction being the other essentials. If the regular physicians of half a century ago had followed the practice of Galen, as described in his works, they would have refreshed their languishing fever patients with cold water as a beverage instead of leaving them to be consumed by the pent-up fires which parched their lips, disorganized their blood, and finally ended their sufferings with their lives. Celsus was proud to boast of employing the bath more frequently and systematically than others had done before his time.

The Emperor Augustus was cured, by the bath, of a disease which had baffled all other remedies.

Testimony of Arabian Physicians.—Although the Arabians are at the present day looked upon, and justly, as a horde of wandering wild-men, a thousand years ago their physicians were among the most learned of the age; and they were as sensible as learned, we judge, for they were most enthusiastic advocates of the efficiency of the bath. Rhazes, one of the most eminent of them, describes a plan of treating small-pox and measles which would scarcely be modified by the most zealous advocate of water treatment at the present day. Avicenna and Meshnes, with others, may be mentioned as holding similar views.

The bath was much used in pestilences by this nation, and was largely employed in Constantinople in the fifteenth century.

Modern Bathing Customs.—Three centuries ago, public vapor baths were very numerous in Paris, being connected with barber shops, as are many baths in this country at the present time. According to Dr. Bell, Paris can still boast of a great number of bathing establishments. He states that in the baths connected with the city hospitals nearly 130,000 thousand baths were administered in a single year to out-door patients. Doubtless those treated in the hospitals were duly washed and steamed as well. This is certainly a very marked contrast with what we see in the hospitals in this country at the present day. Notwithstanding the advances in many other particulars of hospital management, the cuticles of patients are sadly neglected. In some of our largest hospitals, the filthiness of many patients is so great that close proximity to them is absolutely intolerable. Half a dozen of them, placed in a warm room, speedily impart to the air a fetor unequaled by anything but the effluvia arising from a neglected pig-sty. Such neglect is inexcusable.

The Germans of olden time were very fond of bathing, according to their historical records, and during the Middle Ages, when plagued by the leprosy, the national faith in the virtues of the bath was manifested by making it a religious duty. It is related of Charlemagne that he used to hold his court in a huge warm bath. Modern Teutons seem less partial to the bath, having transferred their fondness from *aqua pura* to lager beer.

Although the bath was very freely used in England while the island was occupied by the Romans, who erected commodious baths like those in Rome, the wholesome practice is now sadly neglected by the English people, if we may credit their own writers.

It is a curious fact that the bath seems to be quite generally neglected by the most civilized races, while it is almost universally employed by those less advanced nations, the Russians, Turks, Finlanders, and the inhabitants of Persia, Egypt, Barbary, and Hindostan. The Finlanders make great use of the sweating bath. To nearly every house is attached a small sweat-house, where they subject themselves to a temperature of more than 160° F., often emerging at once into an atmosphere much below freezing, with apparent impunity. The Turkish and Russian baths, similar to which are those in use in Egypt and India, are elsewhere described.

The North American Indians employ the bath for many diseases. They have original and peculiar ways of administering both water and vapor baths. The most common bath among them is the vapor, followed by a plunge into a neighboring stream. They generate the steam by pouring water upon hot stones while they are inclosed in a small, close hut made of mud or skins. The native Mexicans secure a hot-air bath by confining themselves in a brick sweat-house which is heated by a furnace outside. These savages seem to have the most implicit confidence in the efficacy of the bath, always employing it when ill, and with excellent success.

Modern Medical Use of Water.—In the early part of the eighteenth century, a Sicilian named Fra Bernado acquired the title of "cold-water doctor" from his exclusive use of cold water in treating the sick.

At the very beginning of the eighteenth century, Floyer published a history of bathing which contains accounts of many remarkable cures effected by means of the bath, which he recommended as a most efficient cure for numerous diseases.

A Mr. Hancock, a clergyman, published, in 1722, a tract entitled, "Common Water the Best Cure of Fevers." Another writer, in a work entitled, "The Curiosities of Common Water," published in 1723, speaks of water as an "excellent remedy which will perform cures with very little trouble, and without any charge," and "may be truly styled, an universal remedy." Both French and German writers were zealously advocating the use of water as a remedy for many diseases at this same period. Many of the French surgeons had also discovered the immense utility of water in surgery, receiving their first lessons of instruction from an ignorant and superstitious miller, who used water in conjunction with charms.

In the latter part of the last century, Drs. Jackson and Currie each published reports of cases of fever in which they had found the use of the bath a remedy of remarkable efficacy. Dr. Currie obtained many followers for a time, but no very deep impression was made upon the public mind, though his cases were authentic, and were very ably reported.

About the end of the first quarter of the present century, a native of Græfenberg, Prussia, by the name of Priessnitz, met with an accident by which three of his ribs were broken. He treated himself by applications of cold water, and then tried the same remedy upon others in similar cases. His success encouraged him to make further experiments, and though an ignorant peasant, his natural acuteness enabled him to devise various means for applying water to the body, and to suit the application to different diseases. His increasing success attracted numerous patients, and his fame became, in a few years, world-wide. Many of his methods were very rude, and his ignorance of medical science often led him into errors; but he succeeded in restoring to health hundreds of patients whose maladies had been pronounced incurable.

The interest in the new method became so great that numerous other individuals, equally ignorant and possessing less shrewdness, undertook to imitate the German innovator. Some of them were successful, many of them were not; all were alike in committing numerous blunders through ignorance of scientific medicine. But the public attention was called to the utility of water as a remedial agent so forcibly that a powerful impression was produced in its favor. From that time until the present, the use of water has been largely in the hands of unscientific empirics who have advocated it as a specific, and employed it to the exclusion of other remedies in a great degree. This course, together with many other gross errors connected with the practice, has deterred scientific physicians from employing it sufficiently to test its merits, only in a few exceptional instances.

The friends of Priessnitz claimed for him a great discovery ; but as we have seen, he discovered nothing which was not known a century before, if not, indeed, some thousands of years previous. It is doing Priessnitz no injustice to say that he did little or nothing toward establishing principles, but followed, chiefly, a routine method of practice.

Some scientific members of the medical profession have investigated the subject in some degree, however, at various times, and the result has been that at the present day the utility of water is a well-recognized fact, and it is now often prescribed in the standard text-books as an excellent remedy for many diseased conditions. Yet, that there is still a want of appreciation of the remedy is fully attested by the infrequency of its use by the regular profession. This neglect may be due in part to a prejudice which the members of the regular profession have acquired, on account of the quackery which has too often been connected with the use of this remedy. Nevertheless, there is no good reason why an efficient remedial agent should be suffered to receive the stigma which properly attaches only to those who are responsible for its abuse.

REMEDIAL PROPERTIES.

THE value of a drug is judged by its medicinal properties. The more properties it has, and the more powerful its "action," the more valuable it is considered to be. We need not here enter into a discussion of the nature of medicinal properties, since there is no question among scientific physicians, that the medicinal properties—so-called—of drugs, or their effects upon the human system in diseases, are, in general, the result of vital resistance on the part of the system, an attempt to expel or remove the poison, or defend itself against it. Water also possesses remedial properties, some of which are due to vital resistance, while others grow out of the aid which it affords the vital organs by its physical properties. As its value as a curative agent depends upon these properties, it is important to know what they are.

Refrigerant. — Refrigerant or antiphlogistic medicines are used for the purpose of diminishing the heat of the body. The most they can do is to so depress and paralyze the vital forces as to diminish the *production* of animal heat. Water, when applied at a proper temperature—any temperature less than 98°—not only diminishes the production of heat, but removes the superfluous heat by conduction. There is not a drug in the whole materia medica that will diminish the temperature of the body so readily and so efficiently as water. How this is effected, has been previously explained in considering the physiological effects of water.

Sedative.—Drugs, the administration of which is followed by a diminished action of the heart, are termed sedatives. They comprise the most powerful poisons known. Their sedative effects are the result of their poisonous influence upon the heart or the nerve centers controlling it. Water is a much more efficient sedative, and its use is never followed by poisonous effects, as is the use of sedative drugs, the "action" of which is often very uncertain. By the cool or cold bath, the pulse may often be reduced twenty to forty beats in a few minutes.

Tonic.—Water may be used in such a way as to increase the rapidity of the circulation and the temperature very quickly and powerfully. The hot bath is a most efficient stimulant, in the true sense of the word. It will so excite the circulation as to increase the pulse from seventy to one hundred and fifty in fifteen minutes. The tonic effects of a cool bath are well appreciated by all who have ever enjoyed it.

Anodyne.—Certain drugs are called anodyne because they diminish nervous sensibility, thus relieving pain. Water applied in the form of a hot fomentation will not infrequently give relief when every drug has failed. Applied in various other ways, it is very effectual in allaying nervous irritability.

Antispasmodic.—No remedy is so certainly successful in hysterical convulsions as water. In infantile convulsions, its success is also unrivaled. In cramp, and even in puerperal convulsions, its utility has been well demonstrated.

Astringent.—The value of cold water in arresting hemorrhage is well attested by all physicians.

Laxative.—Used in various ways, water is very effectual in producing movement of the bowels, but never occasions those violent and unpleasant symptoms which accompany and succeed the use of purgatives.

Emetic.—In the great majority of cases, no other emetic is needed, and no better can be found.

Eliminative.—Water is a most perfect eliminative. It dissolves the excrementitious and other foreign elements of the blood, and thus materially aids in their elimination. Hence, it is a very useful *diaphoretic*, increasing the action of the skin, and is equally valuable as a *diuretic*, having the same effect upon the kidneys.

Alterative.—For a long period, mercury has been considered as the champion alterative of the materia medica. It must yield the place to wa-

ter, however; for the most it can do is to destroy
the elements of the blood, while water not only
accelerates waste, but increases construction in
the same proportion, according to the experiments of Prof. Liebig.

Derivative.—One of the most important properties of water applications is their powerful derivative effect. No other application, internal or
external, can equal them in efficiency and certainty of action.

There are very few agents which possess so
many remedial properties as water. There are
none which effect so much with so little expense
to the vital powers of the patient. Many drugs
will produce results similar to those obtained by
the use of water, and thus accomplish good, no
doubt; but at the same time, they often work so
much mischief in the system that the evil done
is frequently much greater than the good accomplished. The aim of the faithful physician should
be to accomplish for his patient the greatest
amount of good at the least expense of vitality;
and it is an indisputable fact that in a large number of cases water is just the agent with which
this desirable end can be obtained.

Testimony of Eminent Physicians.—The tes-
timonies of Currie, Jackson, and numerous
other physicians of the last century have already
been quoted in favor of water. There are numerous practitioners of the present day who are

equally favorable to this remedial agent. Perhaps we cannot do better than to quote from the *Health Reformer* the following paragraphs of an abstract report of a paper read before the New York Academy of medicine, by Prof. Austin Flint, M. D., president of the society, the title of the paper being, " The Researches of Currie, and Recent Views Concerning the Use of Cold Water ":—

"Currie employed scientific methods in observing the phenomena of disease. He was one of the first to employ the thermometer in studying disease, and his observations can be received as reliable.

"The use of water externally as a means of reducing the temperature of the body in disease has recently been coming quite prominently into notice. According to Liebermeister, a noted German medical author, Currie was the first to systematize the use of water. His work was published in 1797. Liebermeister, in his recent article on typhoid fever, accords to cold water the first place in importance as an article for reducing the temperature. The use of water for this purpose is at present attracting much attention; and it is safe to predict that *it will soon occupy an important place as a remedial agent.*

"Much harm has been done by the ' rude empiricism ' of Priessnitz, and the various water cures in the country; though much good has also been accomplished by the latter institutions, and they have in a measure prepared the public mind for the general introduction of water as a remedial agent.

"After the publication of the views of Currie in 1797, his method of practice, which was chiefly hydropathic, became quite general, but it was soon nearly forgotten. Trousseau recommended water treatment in scarlatina, and the use of the remedy has continued to be recommended in the text-books; but as a measure of treatment in practice, it has become nearly obsolete. It is, however, obvious that unless we accept the absurd proposition that diseases have changed since Currie's time, the remedy which he recommended so highly must be just as efficient now as then.

"Dr. Currie made use of the cold douche in fevers, applying it vigorously to the patient while in the height of the fever, and continuing it until the temperature became decreased, as indicated by the thermometer and the pulse. He treated seven cases of continued fever by this method at the Liverpool Infirmary. All recovered. In an epidemic of typhoid fever among a regiment of troops, he treated fifty-eight cases, using the cool tepid douche in all but two cases. The latter died. The remaining fifty-six recovered, the disease being greatly shortened in more than half the cases.

"Dr. Currie asserted that, in small-pox, the

use of the bath afforded instant relief to the patient, and caused the disease to assume a benignant form.

"He found the cold bath always effectual in tetanus and convulsions, as also in hysteria.

"In temporary insanity from the use of liquor, this acute observer found that the cold plunge was the most efficient remedy for the worst cases.

"But Dr. Currie's practice was not confined to cold water. He observed that affusion with tepid water was not only a more pleasant application, but that it was even more effectual in reducing unnatural heat than cold water, as it produced no reaction, not being at all stimulating in character.

"With regard to the efficacy of this agent, Dr. Currie stated that by its use in fevers the pulse would be reduced thirty or forty beats, with a corresponding decrease of temperature and almost immediately relief of headache.

"In his second volume, published some six years after his first volume, Dr. Currie declared that although his experience in the use of water, especially in fevers, had been very extensive, he had had only four fatal cases in which water was employed, and had never met with a single evidence of its being in the least degree objectionable or injurious. Neither had he found that it had been thought to be objectionable by those whom he had treated. He details a very interesting account of his treatment of scarlatina in the cases of his two sons, aged, respectively, three and five years. He gave the older, in thirty-two hours, fourteen affusions, varying from cold to tepid. Twelve were found to be sufficient for the younger one. Both became convalescent in three days.

"It was established by Currie that by the use of water the course of typhoid fever may be abbreviated. This is not even claimed for the modern remedies in common use.

"In referring to his own experience in the use of water, Dr. F. remarked, 'The relation of my own experience will of necessity be stated in a few words, as my employment of the remedy has heretofore been much more limited than it will be in the future if my life is spared.' He then related some very interesting cases in which he had employed water as the chief remedy with the most excellent success. He also took occasion to recommend, as one of the best means of applying water in fevers, the wet-sheet pack as employed in the various hydropathic institutions of the country. He had used the continued cold pack in a number of the worst cases of sun-stroke in Bellvue Hospital with marked success. This remedy is still employed there in this class of cases.

"In a case of obstinate remittent fever, which was not in the least benefited by the thorough use of quinia, he employed the cool pack thirty-five times in a week, continuing each application from ten to thirty minutes, and always with great relief to the patient, although he finally died [perhaps from the huge doses of quinine previously given]. He expressed the opinion that if he had employed the pack more thoroughly, making the applications longer and more frequent, the patient might have recovered.

"Currie announced a true theory when he said that *the voice of nature should not be superseded by theories.* He advocated the free use of water as a beverage in febrile diseases [fever] as an important remedial agent. Dr. F. unhesitatingly advanced the belief that the chief benefit derived from the numerous mineral waters so largely used was only that which was due to the properties of pure water. He stated as proof that it was not long since demonstrated by chemical analysis that the only thing peculiar about the water of a certain spring, famous for medicinal virtues, was its remarkable purity. He also suggested the introduction of distilled water for cooking and drinking purposes as a necessary sanitary measure.

"Dr. F. then related a remarkable case of acute inflammation of the kidneys in which the patient exhibited the characteristic symptoms of poisoning from the retention of urea. After other remedies were tried in vain, the patient's life was

saved by the simple administration of water as a
beverage at short intervals. The diuretic effects
of the water soon washed away the poison and
gave immediate relief."

"After the conclusion of the paper, by Dr.
Flint, the venerable Dr. Richards arose and gave
his experience in the use of water. His ideas of
hydropathy were obtained when he has a young
man, from Dr. Currie's works. He adopted the
practice of Dr. C. at that time in an epidemic of
typhoid fever, and with such remarkable success
as to astonish old practitioners. He stated that
he had cured more than one hundred cases of obstinate constipation by simply directing the patient to drink a glass of cold water half an hour
before breakfast, each morning. In one of these
cases the patient had not had a natural passage
from the bowels for a number of years; but he
was effectually cured, by the simple remedy mentioned, in the course of a few months.

"Dr. Loyle gave an interesting resumé of ten
years' experience in the use of water, with uniform success, especially in convulsions and scarlatina. He had employed water alone in about
one hundred cases of acute inflammation of the
kidneys and dropsy after scarlatina, and with
wonderful success in every case. He had found
it equally successful in coma, restoring conscious-
ness when life was apparently extinct. During
the late war, he on one occasion renovated twenty

ambulance loads of exhausted soldiers who had fallen on the march, by the judicious use of water. He recommended water most highly as an excellent diuretic and a capital regulator of the bowels, far superior to 'after-dinner pills.' He commended it also as an efficient remedy for sunstroke and frozen feet.

"The sentiment of the audience—which was wholly composed of medical gentlemen—was shown by the hearty applause with which the remarks of each speaker were received."

We might add much other medical testimony ; but as we could give no higher authority than the distinguished Dr. Flint, who stands at the head of medical practice in America, being author of the standard American text-book on practical medicine, we will not weary the reader with further quotations. The German physicians, as well as German medical works, abound with tributes to the value of water. American medical journals are full of accounts of the beneficial results following its use in fevers and numerous other diseased conditions.

In surgery, the employment of water is rapidly gaining entire precedence. It has replaced nearly all other kinds of dressing for wounds, and its use has saved a valuable limb to many a poor sufferer who must otherwise have submitted to amputation.

In short, wherever it is faithfully and intelligently applied, water is working wonders. Yet it is still little used in comparison with its importance. Especially is its use neglected in chronic diseases. The only reason we have been able to discover for this neglect of a remedy, the merits of which are so well demonstrated and generally acknowledged, is that its use is more troublesome and laborious than the use of drugs. A half-dozen purgative pills are administered much more easily than an enema. The administration of a diaphoretic powder is far more convenient than a pack. A blister is easier to manage than a fomentation. But the true physician, who has at heart the real good of his patient, will not sacrifice the safety or comfort of the latter to his own personal convenience.

ERRORS IN WATER CURE,

MUCH of the prejudice against the use of water in treating disease has grown out of abuses of the remedy, and the putting forward of absurd claims by ignorant persons professing to understand its use. In order to vindicate the character of this powerful curative agent, it is necessary to expose the errors and ignorance of those who have abused it.

"**Cold-Water Doctors.**"—In the early days of the modern water-cure practice, which was very largely introduced by Priessnitz, cold water was the universal remedy. No matter what the nature of the disease, or the condition or temperament of the patient, the remedy was the same. At the establishment of the Græfenberg doctor, ice-cold douches, precipitated from a height of sixteen to eighteen feet, the plunge, directly supplied by the cold mountain springs, and the shower bath of the same temperature, were all administered to patients with little discrimination of modifying circumstances, in rooms unwarmed by artificial heat, even in the depths of the coldest mountain winters. As Græfenberg was the source whence most water doctors of that time drew their knowledge, the same practice was pursued elsewhere. The unreasonableness of such a course was perceived by the more judicious, and thus its influence was prejudicial.

Heroic Treatment.—Such treatment as that described in the preceding paragraph could not result otherwise than disastrously in numerous cases. The evil effects were sometimes seen at once, but more frequently they appeared after periods more or less remote. In some cases, patients were led to drink twenty or thirty glasses of cold water before breakfast, under the absurd doctrine that the evils of a small excess would be cured by greater indulgence. Hundreds of persons adopted the practice of daily bathing in cold water in a cold room, even in the coldest weather. A few even went so far as to spring from their warm beds on the coldest mornings, run to a neighboring brook in a state of nudity, and plunge into its frigid waters through a hole in the ice. So infatuated were these enthusiasts, they really thought they enjoyed this refrigerating process; but, generally, a few years' continuance of it was sufficient to produce such a "sedative" effect upon their systems that some became the victims of consumption and other constitutional diseases, while others were compelled to discontinue the practice from absolute inability to continue it. A few of the more vigorous were enabled to survive this violent treatment without apparent injury for a long time; but those of weaker vital powers soon showed the results of its evil effects.

By such processes, together with the cold sitz bath, the dry pack, and other harsh measures, the patient was sometimes brought to the very verge of the grave.

Strange as it may appear, those who have been the strongest opponents of the use of water, themselves afford the best instances of its excessive use. For instance, in a case of low typhus fever, a "regular" physician ordered the patient, a young woman, to be immersed in cold water for half an hour. The attendants attempted to carry out the prescription, but in a few moments her symptoms became so alarming that the patient was removed from the bath. It will not be considered remarkable that she died. A prominent New·York physician, a professor of practice in one of the largest medical colleges in America, in a report of a case of remittent fever which he had treated with water, said that he administered thirty-five cold packs in a week. The patient died; but the doctor thought that if he had been more thorough in his treatment, giving more packs and longer ones, he would have lived. Another professor, of a rival college in the same city, cited, in a public lecture, a case of pneumonia which was treated hydropathically by a regular physician of note. The patient, while very feeble, was placed in a cold bath. He was taken out shivering, and died an hour afterward. His conclusion was that water was a very hazardous remedy. We would certainly agree with the professor's conclusion if the case cited were an example of the *proper* use of water. In the preceding case, we will not say that the packs were not beneficial; but if they had been thus used by a professed hydropathist, the treatment would have been pronounced decidedly heroic by "regulars."

Crisis.—By the violent processes which have been mentioned, the patient was frequently brought into a condition similar to that produced by the old process of depletion by bleeding, antimony, mercury, and purgatives. Painful skin eruptions, boils, and carbuncles, often covered the whole body. Acute pains racked the body of the patient from head to foot. If he survived this "crisis," he usually got well, which was regarded as an evidence of the salutary effect of the crisis, and so it became an important object to be attained; and the worse a patient felt, the more certain and speedy, he was encouraged to believe, would be his recovery. No account was taken of the immense waste of vital energy during these painful morbid processes.

The use of the abdominal bandage, continued for a long time until an eruption is produced, is another means by which some have sought to effect a cure of their patients. This course is pursued under the belief that the discharge occurring from the surface which thus becomes diseased is a vicarious means of removing impurities from the system—an absurd notion which no one acquainted with the first principles of physiology and surgical pathology could entertain for a moment.

Hydropathic Quacks.—Unfortunately for the reputation of water as a remedy, its use has been largely in the hands of empirics who have used it in a routine manner, and have supposed it to be a cure-all, and the only remedy of any value. At least, such have been the claims made for it. This has served to bring it into disrepute, the disgrace which ought to attach to individuals being applied by an undiscriminating public to the innocent victim of abuse.

Ignorance.—The greatest bane of all has been the ignorance of those who have professed to be qualified to administer water as a remedy understandingly. Priessnitz himself was an ignorant peasant. He was innocent of either anatomical or surgical knowledge. His slight acquaintance with physiology was gathered by cursory observations of patients. Of the effects of water he knew more, studying them with a good degree of acuteness. His lamentable want of knowledge allowed him to fall into many errors. It is related of him that he treated hopeless cases of solid anchylosis of joints just as though they were mere cases of stiffness from rheumatism. Cases of hopeless organic disease, he pronounced curable and submitted to long but unavailing treatment, not knowing the real nature of the disease. A young lady died of what he supposed an internal abscess. No abscess was found, upon which he remarked that "she had too short a neck for long life."

It could be no wonder, then, that the disciples of such a master should be sadly lacking in many of those qualifications essential for a successful physician, no matter what the remedies employed. The most lamentable feature of the matter is that the same ignorance has continued to be, with few exceptions, characteristic of those who have employed water as a remedy; this has been especially disastrous because a man with the native shrewdness and acuteness of perception of Priessnitz has rarely appeared in the ranks of hydropathists.

A Popular Error.—It is a grievous popular error that any one can apply water as skillfully as the most experienced physician, and that its successful use requires no knowledge of the structure and functions of the human body. No doubt this has grown out of another error, perhaps quite as common; viz., that water is so simple a remedy that it will do no harm if it does no good. Such notions have frequently led to most disastrous results. Water, as already shown, is one of the most powerful remedies. And while it is, undoubtedly, far safer in the hands of the uneducated than blisters, purgatives, diuretics, and such agents as opium, chloral, alcohol, and most other drugs, yet it certainly requires careful usage, and the more scientific knowledge the user possesses, the more skillfully will he be able to apply it. It is, furthermore, true that a great majority of ordinary diseases are commonly so void of danger under careful nursing and hygienic management that the application of water is a simple matter which any intelligent mother can perform successfully. A case is related by good authority of a person who fell in apoplexy an hour after taking an excessively hot bath. Another patient became a paralytic from the same cause. Water is a remedy which cannot be safely used by one who has not informed himself of its effects, and of the proper modes of application.

Absurd Claims.—Sensible people have been rightfully disgusted with the claims which have been made by certain pretentious ones for the use of water. One declares that the bath will dissolve out of the body mineral substances which have been taken into it. Another claims to have been able, by the application of fomentations to a rheumatic knee, to extract in regular order the ointments which had previously been successively applied. Numerous other claims equally preposterous might be related, if it were necessary.

They have all tended to excite a feeling of contempt for a means of treating disease which is really worthy of the highest estimation.

Neglect of Other Remedies.—As has been previously remarked, many seem to have forgotten that water is not the only remedy for disease, and not only attempt to cure every disease by its application, but use it to the exclusion of all other remedies. In nearly all cases, sunlight, pure air, rest, exercise, proper food, and other hygienic agencies are quite as important as water. Electricity, too, is a remedy which should not be ignored; and skillful surgery is absolutely indispensable in not a small number of cases. Even drugs are sometimes useful auxiliaries, though, doubtless, infinitely more harm has resulted from the employment of drugs in conjunction with water treatment than from their omission.

Rational Hydropathy leaves room for every other remedy of value. It does not regard water as a specific nor as a panacea, but only as one of the most valuable of numerous excellent remedies. It discards the erroneous and harmful practices of empirics and ignorant charlatans, whether they concern water or other agents, and gives to the aqueous element only its due share of importance.

APPLICATIONS OF WATER.

THE indications which are to be met in the treatment of disease are chiefly those enumerated below; and how admirably they are met by applications of water may be easily demonstrated by following the directions given.

1. Equalization of Circulation. — Disease cannot exist without some disturbance of the circulation. In perfect health each part receives its due share of blood. One of the first indications in disease, then, is to balance the circulation. If an organ contains too much blood, the application of cold water to the part will occasion contraction of the minute vessels of the part, and thus the amount of blood is lessened, as explained more at length in considering the physiological effects of water.

Or, the part may be relieved by the application of warm water in some form to adjacent or remote parts of the body, by which means the surplus blood will be drawn to other parts, thus relieving the suffering organ. Again, if an organ contains too little blood, the opposite course must be pursued. Warm or hot applications are made to the part, while cold applications may be made to other parts if necessary. Very often the two remedies may be advantageously combined, since one part cannot contain too much blood without some other part or parts being deprived of the due proportion, and *vice versa;* so that while a cold application is needed at one part, the opposite is required at another.

2. Regulation of Temperature.—As the condition of the bodily temperature is closely associated with that of the circulation, the two are usually controlled by the same remedies applied in the same manner. A part which contains too much blood has usually, also, too high a degree of heat. The cold application relieves both. If the entire surface of the body is involved, the application must be as extensive as necessary to affect the whole. In general fevers, the admirable adaptation of water to this end is well exhibited. When the temperature of the body rises above 100°, or even above 98°, a cooling bath should be resorted to. It may consist of a simple sponging with water, scarcely below the bodily temperature, an affusion with tepid water, a full bath of a tepid, temperate, or cold temperature, or some other form of cooling application according to the degree of cooling effect desired. Any temperature below 98° will be cooling. In general, it is better to employ a bath only a few degrees below the bodily temperature, as its application will not be followed by an increase of heat, called reaction, which follows a brief application of a cool bath. To obtain the proper cooling effects of a cool or cold bath, it must be continued for some time, from ten minutes to half an hour, at least. The same remark applies also to the application of cool baths for the purpose of equalizing the circulation.

3. Removal of Pain.—Pain is usually dependent upon disturbance of the circulation, being caused by the pressure of overfilled vessels upon the nerves in a confined space. Pain may be relieved by either hot or cold applications. The first object should be to remove the surplus blood, by local cold applications, and remote hot ones. If this plan is not successful, relief will be obtained by a hot local application, which operates by relaxing the surrounding tissues, so that the nerve fibers are relieved from pressure, as well as by quickening the local circulation, and so relieving congestion. The latter method is usually most quickly successful; but it is not so radically curative as the former. Pain dependent on passive congestion will be best relieved by the method next described.

4. To Excite Activity.—Many organs often become torpid or inactive, as the skin and liver, especially. Sometimes the blood-vessels of an organ become relaxed and inactive, passive congestion resulting. No remedy will so readily induce a return of activity to the affected parts as alternate hot and cold applications, continued for some minutes, fifteen to thirty or more. This is one of the best applications for the relief of old pains.

5. Removal of Obstructions.—A very large class of diseases are attributable to obstruction in various organs, caused by the reception of foreign matters into the system, and the accumulation of the natural waste of the tissues. The warm bath, to remove external obstructions, and the internal use of water as a solvent for internal sources of obstruction, are the remedies which will achieve success in nearly all cases. Offending substances in the stomach are readily removed by the water emetic; and hardened accumulations in the large intestine are removed with equal facility by means of the enema.

6. Dilution of the Blood.—In fevers, cholera, and other diseases, the blood often becomes abnormally thickened, dark, and viscid, circulating with difficulty, and not imparting due nourishment to the tissues. Nothing but water can remedy this difficulty. It may be got into the blood by absorption from the skin, if the mucous membrane of the stomach will not absorb it.

7. Influence on the Nervous System.—Finally, it is often important to affect certain organs through their nervous centers. Water, properly applied, will accomplish this also. A fo-

mentation applied to the abdomen will often remove headache, and is an excellent remedy for general nervousness, seeming to affect the whole system, just as does galvanic electricity when applied to the same locality, doubtless through the large nervous ganglia located in that region. Some physicians claim to have obtained peculiar results by the application of heat or cold to the spine. It is said, for example, that cold applied to any portion of the spine will produce an increased circulation in the portion of the body supplied with organic nerves from the part. Hot applications to the spine are said to produce a contrary effect upon corresponding organs. Perhaps there should be still further observations upon this subject before any attempt is made to establish a definite law. It is well known that applications of ice to the spine is an excellent remedy for chorea, and several other nervous diseases.

For general nervous irritability, or nervousness, the *warm* full bath may be applied with uniform success. Neither hot nor cold applications are generally useful in such cases.

Temperature of Baths.—The thermometer is the only accurate measure of temperature ; hence the importance of its use in the administration of baths. Yet the thermometer may be abused. A given temperature may seem warm to one individual and tepid or cool to another. The same difference of sensation will occur in the same individual on different occasions. What seems cool to-day will be thought warm to-morrow. The susceptibility of the body to sensations of heat and cold largely depends upon its condition and the temperature of surrounding objects. In consequence of this physiological fact, it is improper to attempt, as some have done, to fix certain exact temperatures at which baths must be given to all persons under all conditions.

For convenience and perspicuity, the temperatures of baths have been divided into six grades, as given in the following table by Forbes; all who attempt to use the bath according to the directions should carefully learn and preserve the distinctions here made :—

1. Cold Bath,	.	.	.	.	33° to 60° F.
2. Cool,	.	.	.	.	60° " 75°
3. Temperate,	.	.	.	.	75° " 85°
4. Tepid,	.	.	.	.	85° " 92°
5. Warm,	.	.	.	.	92° " 98°
6. Hot,	.	.	.	.	98° "112°

The vapor bath ranges from 98° to 120°; the hot-air or Turkish bath from 100° to 160°, or even higher, though not usefully so.

A bath of any temperature above the natural heat of the body, 98°, is a hot bath. At 32°, water becomes ice ; a bath is very rarely given at this temperature, and then the application should be made to only a small surface. Water at 32°, and even ice and snow, may be usefully employed as topical remedies in local diseases. It will rarely be necessary to employ a full bath at a lower temperature than 65°, which will usually seem very cold to the patient. A temperature from 85° to 95° is the most generally useful for baths which involve a considerable portion of the body, though of course higher temperatures are employed in local applications.

How to Determine the Temperature of a Bath without a Thermometer.—It is often necessary to administer a bath when a thermometer cannot be obtained. In such cases it is customary to test the temperature by placing the hand in the water. This is an unreliable method, however; for the hand becomes, by usage, so obtuse to heat that water which would seem only warm to it would be painfully hot to the body of the patient. To avoid this source of error, it is only necessary to plunge the arm to the elbow into the water, by which means its real temperature will be determined. Water which causes redness of the skin is hot; when it feels simply comfortable, with no special sensation of either heat or cold, it is warm. Slightly cooler than this, it is tepid. When it causes the appearance of goose-flesh, it may be for practical purposes called cool, a still lower degree being cold.

Another Method.—The method about to be described is somewhat more accurate than the preceding, and may be found convenient for facilitating the preparation of a bath of proper quantity as well as temperature, a matter which though simple enough is often quite annoying to inexperienced persons. It is a fact of common knowledge that water boils at 212° F. Boiling water, then, is always of this temperature. Well and spring water, and the water of cisterns in winter, does not vary greatly from 53°. The temperature of well and spring water changes very slightly with the seasons. By combining in proper quantities water of these known temperatures, any required temperature may be produced. Not having seen this method suggested before, we have prepared the following table, which may perhaps be used to advantage in the absence of a thermometer; we advise all to obtain and use a thermometer, however, when it is possible to do so :—

Tem. 53°.			Tem. 212°.				
2 qts.	added to	1 qt.	equals	3 qts.	at	106°
2½ "	"	1 "	"	3½	"	98°
3 "	"	1 "	"	4	"	93°
4 "	"	1 "	"	5	"	85°
5 "	"	1 "	"	6	"	80°
6 "	"	1 "	"	7	"	76°
8 "	"	1 "	"	9	"	71°

When larger quantities are needed, it is only necessary to multiply each of the combining quantities by the same number. For instance, if a gallon and a half of water is needed for a foot bath at 106°, pour into a pail or bath-tub four quarts of fresh well water and then add two quarts of boiling water. If four gallons of water are wanted for a sitz bath at 93° (a very common temperature), pour into the bath-tub three gallons of fresh well or spring water, and add one gallon of boiling water. Thus any required quantity can be obtained at the temperatures given. The cold water should be placed in the vessel first, and there should be no delay in adding the hot water, as it would rapidly lose its heat, and thus make a larger quantity necessary. Determinate measurement is not essential. The cold and hot water may be added alternately in proper proportions, being measured by the same vessel until the requisite quantity is prepared.

RULES FOR BATHING.

The following general rules should be carefully studied and throughly understood by any one who expects to employ the bath. Much injury to health and most of the discredit cast upon the use of water as a remedy have arisen from a disregard of some of them :—

1. A full bath should never be taken within two or three hours after a meal.

2. Such local baths as fomentations, compresses, foot baths, and even sitz baths, may be taken an hour or two after a meal; indeed, compresses and fomentations may be applied almost immediately after a light meal, without injury.

3. Employ the thermometer to determine the

temperature of every bath when possible to do so; if not, employ the other methods described.

4. The temperature of the room during a bath should be 70° to 85°. Invalids require a warmer room than persons in health. Thorough ventilation is an important matter; but draughts must be carefully prevented, by screens of netting placed before openings into the room when necessary.

5. Never apply either very cold or excessively hot treatment to aged or feeble patients. Cold is especially dangerous.

6. Hot baths are rarely useful in health. The warm bath answers all the requirements of cleanliness.

7. Never take a cold bath when exhausted or chilly. A German emperor lost his life by taking a cool bath after a fatiguing march. Alexander came near losing his life in the same manner. Many have been rendered cripples for life by so doing. No harm will result from a cool bath if the body is simply warm, even though it may be in a state of perspiration. Contrary to the common opinion, a considerable degree of heat is the best possible preparation for a cold bath. The Finlanders rush out of their hot ovens— sweat-houses—and roll in the snow, without injury.

8. Cold baths should not be administered during the period of menstruation in females. At

such times, little bathing of any kind is advisable with the exception of a warm or tepid sponge bath, or such treatment as may be advised by a physician.

9. Bath attendants should carefully avoid giving "shocks" to nervous people or to those inclined to apoplexy or affected with heart disease. Shocks are unpleasant and unnecessary for any one.

10. Never apply to the head such treatment as will cause shock, as the sudden cold douche, shower, or spray bath.

11. A light hand bath every morning will be none too frequent to preserve scrupulous bodily cleanliness. More than a week should never be allowed to elapse without a bath with warm water and soap.

12. The best time for treatment—especially cool treatment—is about three hours after breakfast.

13. Always employ for bathing purposes the purest water attainable. Soft water is greatly preferable to hard on many accounts.

14. Those not strong and vigorous should avoid drinking freely of cold water just previous to a bath.

15. The head should always be wet before any bath ; and the feet should be warmed—if not already warm—by a hot foot bath, if necessary.

16. In applying a bath to sick persons, it

should always be made of a temperature agreeable to the feelings.

17. One very important element in the success of a bath is the dexterity of the attendant. The patient should be inspired with confidence both in the bath and in the skill of the attendant. The mind has much to do with the effect of a bath.

18. In general baths, the patient, unless feeble, will derive benefit by assisting himself as much as possible.

19. Patients should receive due attention during a bath, so that they may not feel that they are forgotten. Nervous patients often become very apprehensive on this account. It is also important, in most cases, that a reasonable degree of quietude should be maintained.

20. When any unusual or unexpected symptoms appear during a bath, the patient should be removed at once.

21. In case symptoms of faintness appear, as is sometimes the case in feeble patients, during a hot bath, apply cold water to the head and face, give cool water to drink, lower the temperature of the bath by adding cool water, and place the patient as nearly as possible in a horizontal position.

22. The temperature of a warm or hot bath should always be decreased just before its termination as a precaution against taking cold.

23. In health, a cool or cold bath should be

very brief, lasting not more than one or two minutes. A tepid bath should last not more than ten or fifteen minutes. A warm bath may be continued thirty or forty minutes, or even longer, but nothing could be more absurd than the custom prevailing in some places of prolonging the bath to great length. At Pfeffers and Leuck, in Switzerland, many persons spend the whole day in the water, taking their meals on floating tables, and occupying their time in reading, playing chess, and other games. Some remain in the water as many as sixteen hours out of the twenty-four. Of course, certain baths may be advantageously prolonged in cases of disease; but no intelligent physician will now recommend the antiquated practice which we sometimes see represented by a patient seated in a tub, with an open book in hand.

24. It is of extreme importance that the patient should be carefully dried after any bath. A large sheet is much better for this purpose than a towel. An old linen or cotton sheet is preferable to a new one, being softer. Full directions are given under the heading, " Dry Rubbing-Sheet."

25. A patient should never be left chilly after a bath. Rub until warm.

26. It is equally important that the body should not be left in a state of perspiration, for it will soon become chilly.

27. Patients who are able to do so should exercise a little both before and immediately after a bath to insure thorough reaction.

28. An hour's rest soon after a bath will add to its beneficial effects. It is best to go to bed and cover warm.

29. If a bath is followed by headache and fever, there has been something wrong, either in the kind of bath administered, or in the manner of giving it.

30. Very cold and very hot baths are seldom required. The barbarous practices of half a century ago are now obsolete, or should be, if they are not quite discontinued as yet. No good resulted from them which cannot be attained by milder means, and much harm was occasioned which is avoided by the use of less extreme temperatures.

31. Patients should not be allowed to become dependent on any special form of bath, as an after-dinner fomentation to aid digestion, the abdominal bandage, or any other appliance. Destroy such a habit if it has been formed.

32. Order, cleanliness, dispatch, and a delicate sense of propriety are items which every bath attendant should keep constantly in mind, and which will often contribute in no small degree to success in the use of this agent.

33. Never employ a bath without a definite and legitimate purpose in view. It is somewhat

customary, in many institutions where water is employed, to apply it in a routine way. Many baths are prescribed for the sake of producing variety, or pleasing the patient. A faithful and scientific physician will carefully adapt his remedies to the condition of his patient, and will observe the results. It seems to be a prevalent error that it makes little difference how water is applied, provided the patient is only wet. Warm, hot, tepid, temperate, cool, and cold baths are used indiscriminately.

So, also, the different modes of administering baths of the same temperature are disregarded in many cases. In general, each particular form of bath is especially adapted to the treatment of special conditions, and it is the best test of the proficiency of a physician, in the use of water, to observe whether he recognizes the distinctions between the various kinds of baths, and is able to adapt them to the appropriate conditions.

34. Giving too much treatment is likely to be the error into which the inexperienced will fall, rather than the opposite extreme. Nature cannot be forced to do more than she is capable of doing; and as nature must do the healing, if a cure is accomplished, remedies should be of a helping rather than a crowding or forcing nature. The vitality of patients may be expended uselessly by treatment, for baths excite vital resistance, as well as drugs, a fact which many over-

look. The dangers of over-treatment are not so great as some imagine, however, who take the opposite extreme, and advocate *rest* as the great cure-all. We have seen patients who seemed to be quite monomaniacs on the subject of " rest cure," who needed a good thorough stirring up with useful exercise more than any other kind of treatment.

GENERAL BATHS.

Baths applied to the whole surface of the body are, as we have already seen, among the most powerful means of affecting the human system either in health or disease. Baths of a temperature less than that of the body, 98°, unless of very brief application, uniformly decrease the bodily temperature. That the diminution of temperature is not merely local, being confined to the skin and superficial structures, is shown by the fact that the thermometer indicates a decline of temperature in the interior of the body as well. The bath diminishes the production of heat throughout the whole system, besides abstracting large quantities by its contact with the body, as previously explained. The diminution of temperature continues for hours after the bath, especially in cases in which it was excessively high at the time of administration. Hot baths have, in general, an opposite effect.

SWIMMING.

Swimming is a general bath combined with vigorous exercise, as nearly all baths should be. It is one of the most healthful kinds of exercise, if not continued too long, as it frequently is. The temperature of the water is commonly between 70° and 80° F., which make it a temperate bath. Its effects are not far different from other forms of bath of the same temperature. We have not space to devote to a description of the art, since there are valuable treatises on the subject.

PLUNGE BATH.

The hot baths of the ancient Greeks and Romans were usually followed by a plunge up to the neck in a large basin of water four or five feet deep, and large enough to allow the exercise of swimming. Many hydropathic establishments employ the same bath after packs and sweating baths. A bath of this kind is not always attainable without great expense; and it possesses no particular advantage over other methods of cooling the surface after a warm bath. It is a very severe form of bath when employed at a low temperature. In the days of Priessnitz, it was used at a temperature of 45° or 50°. More harm than good would result from a continuous employment of such treatment. The cool plunge should be of but a very few minutes' duration, and the patient should rub himself vigorously during the bath. In this, as in all other cool baths, the first contact with the water produces chilliness or shock. After two or three minutes, or less, this will be followed by a partial reaction, even while the patient is in the water, accompanied by a feeling of comfortable warmth. This will shortly be again succeeded by a second chill, which is not so likely to be followed by prompt reaction; hence, the patient should always take care to leave the bath before the occurrence of the second chill, if he would avoid unpleasant after-effects.

SPONGE BATH.

The sponge or hand bath is perhaps the simplest and most useful mode of applying water to the surface of the body; for it requires the use of no appliances which every one does not possess, and it can be employed by any one without elaborate preparation, and under almost any circumstances. A great quantity of water is not required; a few quarts are a plenty, and a pint will answer admirably in an emergency. A soft sponge, or a linen or cotton cloth, and one or two soft towels, or a sheet, are the other requisites. The hand may be used in the absence of a cloth or a sponge for applying the water.

The temperature of the bath should not be above 95°, and 90° is generally better. Most people can habitually employ a temperature of

75° or 80° without injury. The use of a much lower temperature is not commonly advisable, and is often productive of great injury.

Begin the bath, as usual, by wetting the head, saturating the hair well. Wash the face, then the neck, chest, shoulders, arms, trunk, and back. Rub vigorously until the skin is red, to prevent chilling; for even when the temperature of the room is nearly equal to that of the body, the rapid evaporation of water from the surface will lower the external temperature very rapidly unless a vigorous circulation is maintained.

After thoroughly bathing the upper portion of the body, turn the attention to the lower portion, continuing the rubbing of the upper parts at brief intervals to prevent chilliness. As soon as the bathing is concluded, envelop the body in a sheet and rub dry, or dry the skin with a towel. When the surface is nearly or quite dried, rub the whole vigorously with the bare hand.

The bath should not be prolonged more than ten or fifteen minutes. Five minutes is sufficient to secure all the benefits of the bath, and even three minutes will suffice for a very good bath.

Persons who chill easily will find it better to bathe only a portion of the body before drying it. Some will even find it necessary to retain a portion of the clothing upon the lower part of the body while bathing and drying the upper part.

Weakly patients may receive this bath with very little disturbance, even in bed. Only a small portion of the body should be uncovered at a time, being bathed, dried, rubbed, and then covered while another part is treated in a similar manner.

The sponge bath may be administered anywhere without danger of soiling the finest carpet, by using care to make the sponge or cloth nearly dry before applying it to the body. A rug may be spread upon the floor as an extra precaution. When used for cleanliness—as it should be daily —a little fine soap should be added two or three times a week, to remove the oleaginous secretion from the skin.

This bath is applicable whenever there is an abnormal degree of bodily heat, and in such cases may be applied every half-hour without injury. It is useful in cases of nervousness and sleeplessness, and, in fact, whenever water is required in any form, it may be used with advantage.

RUBBING WET-SHEET.

This bath is administered in two ways; with the sheet very wet, or dripping, and with it wrung nearly dry. The first method is frequently called the dripping-sheet bath. In giving it, proceed as follows:—

When necessary to prevent injury to the floor or carpet, place upon the floor a large rug or oil-cloth. In the center, place a large wash-tub, in the absence of a more convenient vessel. While the patient is making himself ready for the bath, procure two large cotton sheets. Gather one end of each into folds so that it can be easily and quickly spread out; lay one upon a chair close at hand, and place the other in the tub. At a distance of three or four feet from the tub, place a low stool. Now place in the tub—if a bath at about 93° is desired, and this will be the most usual temperature—half a pailful of fresh well or spring water, and one-third as much boiling water. If a thermometer is at hand it should, of course, be used to test the temperature. After the patient has wet his head, let him step into the tub, facing the assistant, with his arms straight and pressed closely to his sides. Now draw up the wet sheet by its gathered end to its full length; draw out one side quickly, place the corner over one shoulder of the patient, and while holding it in place with one hand, quickly draw 'the remainder of the sheet around him with the other, bringing it up well around the neck, and folding the second corner under the top so as to hold it in place. But a few seconds should be occupied in applying the sheet. Then commence rubbing the patient vigorously with both hands, one upon each side, rubbing to and fro three or four times in each place, passing over the whole body very rapidly, and then repeating the same, to prevent chilling of any part. Coarse, robust, and phlegmatic people may be rubbed with a good deal of severity; but persons with delicate skin and acute sensibilities require gentler manipulation.

After three or four minutes of energetic rubbing, pour over the chest and shoulders a pailful of water four or five degrees cooler than that of the bath, which should be in readiness for instant use. Then rub two or three minutes longer. Now quickly disengage the wet sheet, allowing it to drop into the tub. While the patient is stepping upon the stool, quickly grasp the dry sheet, and by the time he is in place, have him enveloped in it. Rub him dry, passing over the whole body several times in rapid succession, to prevent chilling. Care must be taken that every part is thoroughly dried. The head, armpits, groins, and feet are liable to escape attention. No moisture should be left between the toes. After wiping nearly or quite dry, apply the hand-rubbing, as elsewhere described, using care not to induce perspiration by too vigorous or long-continued rubbing. If the skin should become moist from perspiration after having been once dried, gradually lower the temperature of the room and continue light rubbing until the skin becomes dry and cool before allowing the patient to dress.

Very few baths afford a better opportunity for the display of skill and energy on the part of the attendant than this. Some practice is required to enable one to give it really well.

The other form of rubbing wet-sheet is given in about the same manner, the only difference being that the sheet is wrung before its application, and is re-applied one or more times, according as a milder or more severe form of treatment is required. The douche may be reserved until the sheet is removed the last time.

One precaution especially necessary to be observed in this bath, as well as in all others where a tepid application is succeeded by a cooler one, is frequently overlooked. *The second cooler application should never be made until there is good reaction from the first.*

This is an excellent bath to apply after packs or warm baths which have induced perspiration, as hot-air and vapor baths. It is especially applicable to cases in which there is defective circulation in the extremities, torpid skin and liver, and nervousness. It is of special benefit in cases of debility accompanied by night sweats.

WET-SHEET PACK.

When properly administered, this is one of the most powerful of all water appliances. Some skill is needed to apply it with a uniform degree of success. Two or three comfortables or thick blankets, one woolen blanket, and a large linen or cotton sheet are the articles necessary. It is important to be certain that the sheet is sufficiently large to extend twice around the patient's body. More blankets are required in cool weather and by weak patients. Spread upon a bed or straight lounge the comfortables, one by one, making them even at the top. Over them, spread the woolen blanket, allowing its upper edge to fall an inch or two below that of the last comfortable. Wet the sheet in water of the proper temperature, having gathered the ends so that it can be quickly spread out. Wring so that it will not drip much, place its upper end even with the woolen blanket, and spread it out on each side of the middle sufficiently to allow the patient to lie down upon his back, which he should quickly do, letting his ears come just above the upper border of the sheet, and extending his limbs near together. The patient should then raise his arms, while the attendant draws over one side of the wet sheet, taking care to bring it in contact with as much of the body as possible, bringing it closely up beneath the arms, and pressing it down between the limbs so as to make it come in contact with both sides of them. Tuck the edge tightly under the patient on the opposite side, using care not to include the other edge of the sheet. Now let the patient clasp his hands across his chest, and then bring up the other side of the sheet. Grasp it by its upper corner with one hand, drawing it down over the shoulder and

lengthwise of the body; then place the other
hand upon the covered shoulder, holding the
sheet firmly in place while the corner is carried
upward upon the opposite side and tucked under
the shoulder, thus drawing the upper edge of
the sheet well up under the chin. Tuck the edge
of the sheet under the body, carefully enveloping
the feet. Then bring over each side of the blanket and comfortables in the manner last described,
being very careful to exclude all air at the neck,
and allowing the blankets to extend below the
feet so that they can be folded under.

It is not desirable that the patient should be
bound as tightly as a mummy. All that is necessary is the exclusion of air, and as the neck
and feet are the points at which it is most likely
to enter, these parts should receive particular attention, as directed. If too tightly bound, the
patient will be more likely to be nervous than if
allowed some freedom. The application of the
wet sheet should be made in a few seconds, as it
cools very rapidly when spread out. The first
blanket should be brought over the patient as
soon as possible. If the feet are not warm, a hot
foot bath should be taken before the pack. If
they become cool in the pack, hot jugs, bricks, or
stones should be applied to them. If the patient
does not become comfortably warm in a few minutes—ten or fifteen at most—more blankets
should be added, and, if necessary, dry heat should

be applied to the sides. If he still remains chilly, he should be promptly removed and placed in a warm bath, or vigorously rubbed with a dry sheet and then placed in a dry pack. The head should be kept cool by frequent wetting while the patient is in the bath. If a compress is applied, it should be often renewed.

The temperature of the pack must depend upon the condition of the patient, being determined by principles elsewhere explained. A woolen sheet is better for the administration of a hot pack than one of cotton or linen. The cold pack is very rarely required. The usual temperature for this bath should be about 92°. It is proper to wet the sheet in water of about 100°, as it will be cooled several degrees while being applied.

The duration of the pack should be carefully regulated by the condition of the patient, the effects desired, and the immediate effects produced. If the patient becomes very nervous, or sweats excessively, or becomes faint, or has other seriously unpleasant or dangerous symptoms, he should be removed from the pack at once if he has not been more than ten minutes in it. Ordinarily, the pack may continue thirty to forty-five minutes. If the patient sleeps naturally, he may remain in the pack a full hour if strong, or even longer in many cases. In fevers, short packs, frequently repeated, are more beneficial than long ones fewer in number.

The pack should be followed by the spray, the sponge bath, the douche, or the rubbing wet-sheet. It is a powerful remedy, and should not be used to excess in chronic diseases; it has been much abused in this way. Its depurating effects are really wonderful. The increased action of the skin, together with determination of blood to that part, is so great that poisons long hidden in the system are brought out and eliminated. The odor of a sheet recently used in packing a gross person is often intolerable. If the patient be a tobacco-user, the sheet will be reeking with the odor of nicotine. Many times, the sheet will be actually discolored with the impurities withdrawn from the body.

The applications of the pack in treating disease are very numerous. In almost all acute diseases accompanied by general febrile disturbance, and in nearly all chronic diseases, it is a most helpful remedy if rightly managed. It is an admirable remedy for nervousness, skin diseases, and irritations of the mucous membrane. The warm pack is a remedy worth more in the treatment of children's diseases than all the drugs in the materia medica, as many physicians have proved. It is a most successful application in convulsions.

SHOWER PACK.

In many cases of fever in which the temperature rises so high as to produce delirium, the ordinary pack does not seem to be sufficiently powerful to fully control the excessive heat. In such cases, the shower pack is found of great service; it is thus used in Bellevue Hospital, New York :—

A rubber blanket is placed upon an ordinary mattress. Upon this, the patient is placed, enveloped in a wet sheet, as in the ordinary pack. Instead of being covered with blankets, however, he is left exposed to the air, so that the powerful cooling effects of evaporation may be obtained. As the sheet becomes warmed by the heat of the body, cool water is showered upon it from a sprinkler or watering-pot. The bath is continued thus until the temperature of the patient, as indicated by the thermometer, is sufficiently diminished.

This bath, combining as it does the cooling effects of cool water and of evaporation, is the most powerful refrigerant that can be employed; yet it is perfectly safe when judiciously used, being only applied in cases of extreme urgency on account of the high temperature.

Some practice opening the ordinary pack at intervals, and sprinkling cool water upon the patient, thus obtaining, in some degree, the prolonged cooling effect. The pack must be studied well to enable one to apply it with skill, and certainty of success.

DRY-SHEET PACK.

Though this can hardly be called a bath at its commencement, it really becomes a wet-sheet pack before its termination. Its application differs from that of the wet-sheet pack in that the patient is wrapped in woolen blankets instead of the wet sheet. The object of this treatment is to produce perspiration, which may be encouraged by drinking either cold or hot drinks in considerable quantity, and by the application of dry artificial heat to the feet and sides. It is a very severe form of treatment, and is now seldom practiced. Many years ago, patients at hydropathic establishments were often kept for several hours in the dry pack, smothered beneath loads of comfortables, blankets, and feather-beds. If cautiously employed, it is occasionally useful in "breaking the chills," in fever and ague. It should be administered about half an hour before the time for the beginning of the chill, if required for this purpose.

The several varieties of local packs are described under the head of Local Baths.

FULL BATH.

For this bath a tub is required the length of the body, about eighteen inches deep, two feet wide at the top, and preferably, six inches narrower at the bottom. It is better to have the end intended for the head a little elevated,

Place in the tub sufficient water so that the patient will be entirely covered, with the exception of the head, when he lies upon his back. During the bath, the body should be vigorously rubbed by the bather or an attendant, or both, particular pains being taken to knead and manipulate the abdomen, in a gentle, but thorough manner. The temperature of the bath, when taken for cleanliness, or for its soothing effects, should be not more than 95°, and it should be cooled down to about 85° before the conclusion of the bath, by the addition of cool water.

Every family ought to possess conveniences for this bath. Indeed, it is now found in every well-regulated modern house in our large cities. It is not so expensive but that any one can possess it. Portable baths of rubber can be obtained which are worth many times their cost. A cheap bath can be constructed of duck well oiled or covered with paint and suspended from a frame; but it will be quite unsatisfactory, not being perfectly water-tight, as such a bath should be for family use. A stationary bath may be made of wood, of the dimensions given, and lined with lead or zinc. There should be an opening in the lower end for withdrawing the water.

The full bath is one of the most refreshing of all baths, being also one of the most pleasant. Employed at a low temperature, it is a powerful means of reducing excessive heat in fevers. The hot full bath very promptly relieves the pains of acute rheumatism, and is almost a specific for colds, if taken just before retiring. Very hot and very cold temperatures are quite hazardous with this bath, since it involves so large a portion of the body. Such extremes are rarely useful in any case, and should not be used except under the eye of a physician.

HALF BATH.

The half bath is much the same as the full bath. A smaller tub is required, as the bather sits upright with his limbs extended. The water should be at least a foot deep. During the bath, the body should be well rubbed, and water should be poured over the upper portion of the body. Its general effects are nearly the same as those of the full bath, and it may be used for the same general purposes. A little more vigorous rubbing is required to prevent chilling, as so large a portion of the body is exposed. It affords a better opportunity for stirring up the bowels and abdominal viscera by shaking, percussing, and kneading the abdomen.

SHALLOW BATH.

Of this bath there are two varieties; *sitting shallow* and *standing shallow*.

Sitting shallow differs from the half bath in employing less water, and being much more vigorous. Its effects and uses are about the same. The bather should rub his limbs and the front portion of his body while the attendant pours water over his chest and shoulders, and rubs vigorously his back and sides. A person can take the bath very well alone by using a rather long coarse towel which can be drawn back and forth across the back by grasping one end with each hand. It is a very valuable means of applying water, and is in constant requisition in the hydropathic establishments. From 85° to 90° is the proper temperature for this bath. It may be used at a lower temperature in fever cases. At Bellevue Hospital it is applied at about 70° in such cases, and is administered whenever the temperature exceeds 103°. To avoid the shock of a cool bath, it may be commenced at a temperature little below blood-heat and then gradually cooled by the addition of cool water until the desired temperature is reached. The reduction of the temperature obtained by this means fully equals that obtained by the sudden application of cold, and the shock and subsequent reaction are prevented. This applies equally to all cool baths as well as the cool shallow bath.

The duration of the bath may be from one to thirty minutes. Ten or fifteen minutes will be the usual extent.

The Standing Shallow is in some cases preferred by some to the preceding. The patient stands erect in a varying depth of water—from six inches to one or two feet being employed—while his body is vigorously rubbed by one or two assistants, water being poured upon the chest and shoulders at brief intervals. It is a very enlivening bath.

The shallow bath should be completed by a pail douche at a temperature three or four degrees lower than that of the bath.

AFFUSION.

This consists simply in pouring water over the body of the patient, who may be sitting or standing in a bath-tub. It is a very efficient bath for reducing unnatural heat. This mode of treatment was used by Hippocrates, Galen, and other ancient physicians. In the last century, Currie, Jackson, and many others used it with great success in scarlatina. It is a sovereign remedy for delirium tremens, sun-stroke, hysteria, and sometimes of acute mania, when applied of the proper temperature.

PAIL DOUCHE.

This bath scarcely differs from the preceding. It consists in the dashing of one or more pailfuls of water upon the body of the bather by an assistant. By means of a proper arrangement, the bather can administer the bath himself. For this purpose, a pail or other vessel filled with water may be suspended or supported above the head of the bather in such a way that it can be quickly upset by drawing upon a string attached to the side. The stream should fall upon the shoulders, chest, back, or hips, but not upon the head or over the region of the stomach. This bath may be applied after any warm bath, and should be a little cooler than the bath which precedes it. Whether taken alone or after another bath, it should always be followed by vigorous rubbing.

CATARACT DOUCHE.

This is a modification of the douche bath in which a broad sheet of water is allowed to fall upon the body of the bather. The force of the bath depends upon the height from which the water falls, and should be regulated according to the strength of the patient. Almost any one will bear a fall of three or four feet. When the height of the bath cannot be easily modified, it should be of such an altitude as to be well borne by the feeblest patients; the more vigorous can increase its effects by subjecting themselves to it for a longer time.

The observations made relating to the application of the pail douche, apply equally well to this bath.

HOSE DOUCHE.

In this bath, water under pressure is thrown upon the patient from a hose, through a small nozzle. The bather turns his body while the attendant directs the stream upon different parts. It is a less pleasant bath than the spray or other forms of douche. Its general effects are the same as those of the baths mentioned.

SHOWER BATH.

This bath is simply an imitation of rain. Water is allowed to fall upon the body after being divided into a number of small streams by passing through a vessel with a perforated bottom. Its effects depend upon the size of the streams and the height from which they fall, together with the temperature of the bath and its duration. Although formerly much employed in water-cure establishments, this bath is now little used, because its place is supplied by other more convenient ones which produce the same results, as the spray and douche. The best manner of administering it is to commence the application with tepid water, and gradually cool it. The temperature may range from 70° to 92°. The water should not usually be allowed to fall upon the head, but should be received first upon the hands and arms, then upon the feet and limbs, and afterward upon the back and shoulders, the body being well rubbed during the application.

The cold shower bath, formerly so common almost everywhere, has been productive of much injury by its indiscriminate use, and has brought much reproach upon the use of water as a curative agent. None but the most vigorous can enjoy the bath at a lower temperature than 70°, and no advantage is gained by its employment at a lower temperature than that, while considerable harm may be done in many cases.

SPRAY BATH.

This bath consists in a number of fine streams of water thrown upon the bather, with considerable force. It may be produced by connecting a hose with spray attachment to a force-pump or reservoir from which to obtain water under a sufficient pressure. The best form of attachment consists of a hollow double-convex brass or copper piece, one side of which is perforated with fine holes, the other side carrying a rim for attachment to the hose. It is preferable to have an arrangement by which the temperature may be readily and gradually changed from warm or tepid to cool without interrupting the bath. In the absence of a proper spray attachment, the apparatus elsewhere described for the hose douche may be made to answer a very good purpose, the stream being broken by placing the thumb or finger over the nozzle in such a way as to partially obstruct the flow.

This is an excellent bath to follow the pack, vapor bath, hot-air bath, sitz bath, or any other general bath which induces perspiration. It is very agreeable to most persons, and can be applied to feeble patients who would be unable to take any more severe form of treatment. The alternate hot and cold spray is very successful as a means of reducing local inflammations. The warm bath is very grateful and soothing to swollen and rheumatic joints; in gout, also, and illy defined, wandering pains, it is an admirable remedy. It is very successful, also, in the treatment of tumors, abscesses, and chronic ulcers, when thoroughly applied.

LOCAL BATHS.

'The use of water as a local application is not less important, and is much more varied, than its general application. There is no other topical remedy which will produce such a variety of effects and such prompt results. In removing local congestions, subduing local inflammations, allaying circumscribed pain, and restoring activity to inactive parts, the appropriate applications of water give results which afford both physician and patient a degree of satisfaction which no other single remedy can rival, even electricity, an agent of acknowledged power, not being excepted.

SITZ BATH.

The sitz bath, also known as the hip bath, is one of the most useful baths employed in hydropathic treatment. Its utility was fully recognized by the earlier practitioners, who sometimes kept their patients so long in the bath that they became almost literally water-soaked, and were so numb from the long-continued application of cold water as to possess almost no external sensibility. It is said that in some cases the skin could be rubbed off in the attempts to obtain reaction, without the patient's knowledge.

For this bath a common tub may be used, by placing a support under one edge to elevate it two or three inches; but it is better to use a tub made for the purpose, which should have the back raised eight or ten inches higher than the front, to support the back, the sides sloping gradually so as to support the arms of the bather. The bottom should be elevated two or three inches. The depth in front should be about the same as that of a common wash-tub.

Enough water is required to cover the hips and extend a little way up the abdomen; four to six gallons will suffice. Any temperature may be employed, being suited to the condition of the patient. The duration of the bath will also vary according to circumstances. A short cool bath is tonic in its effects, like all short cool applications; a more prolonged one is a powerful sedative.

The hot sitz is very exciting in its effects if long continued. The warm bath is relaxing. The hips and trunk should be well rubbed during the bath by the patient or an attendant. The bather should be covered with a sheet or blanket during the bath. If it is desirable to produce sweating, several blankets may be used.

The sitz bath should seldom be taken either very hot or extremely cold. A very good plan for administering it, and one which will be applicable to most cases, is this: Begin the bath at 92° or 93°. If a thermometer is not at hand, pour into the bath-tub three gallons of fresh well or spring water, and then add one gallon of *boiling* water. This will give the desired temperature. After the patient has been in the bath ten minutes, cool it down to 85°, which may be done by adding a gallon of well water. Continue the bath five minutes longer, then administer a pail douche or spray, at about 85°, and wipe dry, as directed after a rubbing wet-sheet.

The sitz bath is useful for chronic congestions of the abdominal and pelvic viscera, diarrhea, piles, dysentery, constipation, uterine diseases, and genital and urinary disorders. In treating female diseases it is an indispensable remedy. It is very valuable in various nervous affections, especially those which immediately involve the brain.

There is no better remedy for a cold than a

very warm sitz bath taken while fasting, and just before retiring. It should be continued until gentle perspiration is induced.

The sitz may be converted into a general bath by rubbing the whole body with the wet hand while in the bath, and may thus be made to answer the purposes of the half and shallow baths.

LEG BATH.

For this bath a vessel deep enough to receive the limbs to the middle of the thighs is required. The bath may be taken at any desired temperature; but it is usually employed somewhat cooler than baths which involve the trunk of the body. It is a powerfully derivative bath, and is found very useful to prevent wakefulness in nervous persons, and to relieve cerebral congestion in epileptic patients. It is especially applicable to chronic ulcers of the leg, swollen knees and ankles, and limbs which have suffered by exposure to severe cold. It gives much relief in gout; there is no danger of causing a metastasis of the disease by the application of this bath.

FOOT BATH.

Any vessel sufficiently large to receive the feet, and enough water to cover them to the ankles, is suitable for this bath. The feet should be rubbed during the bath. If the temperature is cool, only an inch or two of water should be employed.

The *walking foot bath* is an excellent remedy for cold feet. It consists in walking in shallow water five or ten minutes.

The alternate hot-and-cold *foot bath* is another valuable remedy for cold feet, and is a certain remedy for chilblains. It is given thus: Place the feet in hot water—100° to 110°—three or four minutes. Then withdraw them and plunge them quickly into a bath of cold water—60° or less. After two or three minutes, restore them to the hot bath. Thus alternate three or four times, and conclude by dipping the feet quickly into cold water and wiping dry. This bath produces most powerful reaction.

The foot bath is applicable in the treatment of headache, neuralgia, toothache, catarrh, congestion of abdominal and pelvic organs, colds, and cold feet. It is very useful as a preparatory for other baths, and as an accompaniment of other local applications.

HALF PACK.

This bath is given in the same manner as the wet-sheet pack, except that the wet sheet extends only from the armpits to the hips. The blankets are wrapped about the patient in the manner described for the full pack. All the precautions given in connection with the description of that bath are applicable to this.

This bath is frequently employed in cases of

patients who are too feeble to bear the full pack, or as a preparatory treatment for that bath. It is much milder than the full pack, and is usually more agreeable to the patient, as it does not confine him so closely. It is a very useful remedy in all inflammations of the abdominal organs, gastralgia, pleurisy, acute brochitis, croup, and pneumonia. When a hot application is required, it is well to use a woolen sheet instead of a cotton one. It requires the same after-treatment as the full pack.

CHEST PACK.

This application is made in the same manner as the half pack, allowing the wet sheet to extend only from the armpits to the navel. It is especially applicable to diseases of the chest. The general directions for the full and the half pack apply to it. It is a very mild application.

LEG PACK.

The pack may be applied to the legs with great advantage in cases of habitual coldness of the feet and limbs or knees. The same principles mentioned in relation to other packs apply to this. The application should be made either cool or cold, and should extend from the hips downward. It should continue from half an hour to an hour and a half.

CHEST WRAPPER.

This consists of a jacket made something like a vest, reaching from the neck to a little below the navel. It should be made of double thicknesses of soft toweling. To protect the garments or bedding from moisture, it should be covered with another jacket made like it but a little larger. In applying it, the wrapper should be wet in tepid water, and should then be applied as snugly as consistent with the comfort of the wearer. It should be re-applied every two or three hours, as it becomes dry.

If properly managed, the chest wrapper is a valuable remedy; but it has been greatly abused. It should not be worn more than a week without intermission. The practice of some in continuing it until it produces an eruption of the skin, and even longer—to promote a discharge—under the idea that a vicarious elimination is thus performed, is highly reprehensible, and has no sound physiological principle to support it. Such treatment is damaging to the skin, and does the patient no good in any way. The better plan is to allow the wrapper to be worn during the night, but omitted during the daytime. If worn during the day, it should be changed often, and should be removed so soon as the patient becomes chilly. Whenever removed, the surface of the skin should be washed or sponged with cool or tepid water. Feeble patients with defective circulation should wear the wrapper only while walking or riding on horseback.

This appliance may be profitably employed in a large number of chronic diseases. In chronic bronchitis, pleurisy, pleurodynia, asthma, and the early stages of consumption, it gives relief.

WET GIRDLE.

This was a favorite remedy with the early German hydropathists, and it is a very useful appliance when properly employed, though it has been much abused by excessive use, as in the case of the chest wrapper. To apply it well, a coarse towel about three yards long is the most convenient for use. Wet one-half of this, in tepid water, wring it until it will not drip, and apply it to the abdomen, placing one end at the side, and bringing it across the front first, so that two thicknesses of the wet portion will cover the abdomen. After winding the whole tightly around the body, fasten the end securely. The remarks made in reference to the wearing of the chest wrapper apply with equal force to the wet girdle. For feeble patients it is better to wet only that portion of the towel which covers the abdomen.

This a very efficient remedy for constipation, chronic diarrhea, and most other intestinal disorders. It is equally valuable in dyspepsia, torpid liver, enlarged spleen, and uterine derangements.

ASCENDING DOUCHE.

This modification of the douche is simply an ascending instead of a descending stream. It can be readily managed by constructing a reservoir in such position as to give the water ten or twelve feet fall, when the requisite force cannot be more easily secured. The water is conducted through a hose, and is allowed to issue through a nozzle near the floor. The patient sits or lies just over the nozzle, and a few inches above it.

This is a valuable remedy in treating piles, prolapsus of the bowels or uterus, and constipation.

DROP BATH.

In applying this bath, a vessel with a small opening in the bottom is elevated to a considerable height, water placed in it being allowed to drop upon the part to be treated. The aperture in the vessel should be only sufficiently large to give egress to a single drop at a time. The bath may also be given by placing in an elevated vessel one end of a skein of cotton yarn, the other being allowed to fall over the edge of the vessel and hang below it. By capillary attraction the water will be drawn up into the yarn and will drop off at the lower end very slowly.

This is a very convenient way of applying water where its cooling effects are required for a considerable length of time, as in wounds, bruises, sprains, and similar cases. It will "keep down inflammation " in a wonderful manner. It is not commonly necessary that the water should be very cold, as evaporation will keep the part sufficiently cool in most cases.

ARM BATH.

This is simply holding the arm in water of proper temperature. It is extremely useful in such painful affections as felons, sprains, and nearly all injuries of the hand and arm. Ulcers and acute and chronic skin diseases of the hands and arm are usually benefited by this bath. If cold water is painful, its application should be preceded by that of hot water, or alternated with it. Cold hands should be frequently rubbed in cool water, and alternately immersed for a few minutes each in hot and cold water. In case of painful felons, the arm must be immersed to the elbow to relieve the pain, although the disease is only in the finger.

HEAD BATH.

The patient should lie upon his back, resting his head in a shallow basin of cool water. The attendant should bathe the forehead, face, and temples during the bath. The bath may be continued until the heat is removed or lessened.

The pouring head bath is often preferable to the preceding. The patient should lie upon a bed or sofa, face downward, allowing his head to extend outward over a tub or other wide vessel, while the water is poured upon the head from a little height, by an assistant. The water may be either hot or cold, according to existing conditions. Very cold water is not usually advisable, as its application soon becomes painful, and produces powerful reaction. It should be tepid or temperate. Some cases require very hot water for a few minutes, followed by a slight affusion of tepid water.

In hysteria, epilepsy, apoplexy, sun-stroke, acute mania, delirium tremens, and cerebral congestion from any cause, the head bath is a promptly efficacious remedy.

EYE BATH.

Water may be applied to the eye in various ways. A convenient method when only a brief application is necessary, is to lave the eye with water dipped by the hand. A gentle spray may be applied, or the eyes may be opened and closed in water, thus bringing them freely in contact with the element. Small glass cups made for the purpose may be filled with water and placed over the eye, the water being frequently changed ; or wet cloths may be laid upon them.

In applying water to the eye, it is important to be able to first distinguish the exact nature of the difficulty, as much damage may otherwise be done by a wrong application. As a general rule, inflammations of the conjunctiva and *external* structures of the eye require *cool* or *cold* applications, while inflammations of the cornea, iris, and other *internal* structures, require *hot* applications. This rule is often violated in hydropathic establishments through ignorance of the structure and diseases of the eye.

Cool applications are best made by laying upon the eyes thin folds of linen cloth wet in cold water. Not more than two or three thicknesses should be used, as a thick compress soon becomes warm, while a thin one is kept cool for a longer time by evaporation. The compress should be changed every five minutes, at least, when there is much inflammation. The fomentation is as good as any method of applying hot water to the eyes. The application, when hot, should be as hot as the patient can well bear. If it affords relief, continue half an hour or more; if it increases the pain, desist at once. The same may be said of cold applications also.

Alternate hot and cold applications will give most relief in some cases. After a hot application, a slightly cooler one should always be applied for a few minutes.

A little milk, quince-seed mucilage, or other bland substance, added to the water, makes it more agreeable to the eye in bathing it.

The eye bath is applicable in all inflammations and injuries of the eye, and is infinitely superior to all other eye washes.

Daily bathing the eyes in tepid water is a good practice for those who use them much in reading, writing, or other work requiring close attention. Many eyes are ruined by neglect and maltreatment.

EAR BATH.

Water applications are made to the ear by means of fomentations, compresses, the douche, or the spray. Compresses and fomentations are useful in inflammations of the structures of the ear, including abscesses which often form in the walls of the external canal. Alternate hot and cold applications are useful in causing the absorption of inflammatory deposits, and thus restoring the hearing. The douche, administered with the fountain syringe, is a valuable means of removing foreign bodies and insects. The warm douche has proved very serviceable in restoring the hearing by removing hardened ear-wax. In administering the douche, the head should be inclined over a basin, while the stream of water is allowed to issue from the nozzle held close to the external opening of the ear. Violent syringing of the ear should never be practiced, as it may occasion irreparable injury.

NOSE BATH.

This bath is administered either by drawing water into the nose while the mouth is closed, or by injecting it by means of a fountain syringe.

Great care should always be exercised to apply the water gently, as a forcible application will cause pain and irritation. Injection should never be practiced with a piston syringe, as there is liability of forcing the water into the Eustachian canals and producing deafness. The temperature of the water should be warm or tepid for most applications.

Much benefit may be derived by the proper use of this bath in case of acute or chronic catarrh. The addition of a slight portion of salt to the water does no harm, and a slightly saline fluid is sometimes less unpleasant than pure water, probably because it is more nearly like the mucous secretion of the nasal mucous membrane. Drawing cold water into the nose is sometimes recommended for hemorrhage from the nose; but it is of doubtful utility, because the application cannot be continuous, and transient applications of cold water are always followed by an afflux of blood to the part so exposed. There are better remedies for nose-bleed.

COMPRESSES.

The compress is a wet cloth or bandage applied to a part. The object may be to cool the part under treatment, or to retain heat. The compress may be used with equal success for either purpose. When the part is to be cooled, a compress composed of several folds should be wet in cool, cold, or iced water, as required, and placed upon the part after being wrung so it will not drip. It should be changed as often as *every five minutes.* This is often neglected to the injury of the patient. A very cold compress may be prepared by placing snow or pounded ice between the folds of the compress. This will not need renewal so frequently; but its effects must be carefully watched, as injury may be done by neglect. In applying cold to such delicate parts as the eye, a very thin compress is better. It should be renewed once in five minutes, at least.

When accumulated warmth is required, a thick compress is applied, being wrung out of tepid water, and covered with a dry cloth to exclude the air. Soft, dry flannel is an excellent covering. Rubber or oiled silk may be employed when the compress is not to be retained more than a few hours; but if it is to be worn continuously, they will be injurious, as they are impervious to air and thus interfere with the function of the skin. The effects of a compress thus applied are identical with those of the poultice, and the application is a much more cleanly one.

Compresses are applicable in all cases in which poultices are commonly used. They may replace the old-fashioned plasters with profit and comfort to the wearer. The wet-sheet pack, half pack chest pack and wrapper, leg pack, and wet girdle are all large compresses.

When applied continuously in the same place for a long time, the compress occasions a considerable eruption of the skin, and sometimes boils and carbuncles. There is no particular advantage in these eruptions, and they sometimes do much harm by producing a great degree of general irritation. The notion that they purify the system, though a very popular one, has really a very slight foundation. The discharge is largely made up of elements which would be of great utility if retained in the system, and the amount of foul matter eliminated in this way is certainly infinitesimal compared with the amount thrown off by a few inches of healthy skin. The skin can always do more and better work when healthy than when diseased. The eruptions are no doubt due to debility of the skin, produced by a too long continuance of the very abnormal conditions supplied by the compress. Yet, strange as it may appear, there are those claiming to be physicians who directly aim to produce inflamed and irritated surfaces by the continuation of the compress for months and even years.

The *wet head cap* is a compress made to fit the head. It should consist of several thicknesses of cotton or linen cloth, so as to retain moisture for some time. It is a good temporary appliance in diseases of the scalp, and for headache; but it should never be worn continuously for the purpose of relieving congestion, as it will have an effect just the opposite of that desired. In eczema of the scalp it may be worn until the disease is cured, being frequently rewetted. It is an excellent means of preventing sun-stroke and other effects of heat when worn beneath the hat in summer; but even for this purpose its use should be temporary, the cap being worn only during the hotter portion of the day.

FOMENTATIONS.

The fomentation is a local application analogous to such general appliances as the hot pack, vapor bath, and hot-air bath. It consists in the application of a cloth wet in hot water. It may be considered as a hot compress. Fold a soft *flannel* cloth twice, so that it will be of three or four thicknesses. Lay it in a basin, pour boiling water upon it, and wring it dry by folding it in a dry towel. Or, if only one end of the cloth is wet, it may be wrung by folding the dry portion outside of the wet; in wringing, the whole will become equally wet. Apply it to the patient as hot as it can be borne. The second application can usually be made much hotter than the first. Frequently dipping the hands in cold water will enable the attendant to wring the cloth much hotter than he would otherwise be able to do. The most convenient way is to heat the cloths in a steamer; by this means they are made as hot as boiling water, and yet they are more easily handled, not being saturated with water. When no hot water is at hand, a fomentation may, in an emergency, be quickly prepared by wetting the flannel in cool water, wringing it as dry as desired, folding it between the leaves of a newspaper, and laying it upon the top of the stove, or holding it smoothly against the side. The paper prevents the cloth from becoming soiled, the water protects the paper from burning, and the steam generated quickly heats the cloth to boiling heat. For a long fomentation, the heat may be made continuous by applying over the wet cloth a hot brick or slab of soapstone.

The hot cloths should be re-applied once in five minutes. Two cloths should be employed, so that the second may be applied the moment the first is removed. To retain the heat, a dry flannel, rubber, or oil-cloth should be placed over the fomentation. The application may be continued from ten minutes to half an hour, or longer in special cases. This appliance is very powerful, and should not be employed to excess. Alternate hot and cold fomentations are frequently more efficient than the continuous fomentation. Hot applications should always be followed by a cool or tepid compress for four or five minutes, at least.

The uses of the fomentation are very numerous. It is indicated whenever there is local pain without excessive heat, or evidences of acute inflammation. Local congestions, neuralgia, toothache, pleurisy, pleurodynia, and most local pains vanish beneath its potent influence as if by magic. For indigestion, colic, constipation, torpid liver, dysmenorrhea, and rheumatic pains, it is a remedy of great power, and is used with almost uniform success. In relieving sick headache by application to the head, neck, and stomach, its efficiency is unrivaled.

When applied to the head for some time without intermission, it will often occasion faintness; hence, a cooler application should be made after the use of the hot cloths for fifteen or twenty minutes.

If the applications must be continued for a long time, it is well in most cases to apply them at a temperature slightly lower than when they are to be used for only a few minutes.

This remedy may well replace the blisters, plasters, cataplasms, scarifications, rubefacients, and other irritating measures so long used for relieving pain, local congestions, and inflammations.

REFRIGERANT APPLICATIONS.

A freezing mixture which will reduce the temperature to 4° is made by mixing equal parts of salt and pounded ice. The ice and salt should be stirred together very quickly and applied at once to the part to be frozen. Two parts of dry snow and one of salt make an equally good mixture. Freezing is more conveniently performed by the rapid evaporation of ether or rhigoline.

Freezing is a useful process in numerous cases. By its use, excresences—as warts, wens, and polypi —fibrous tumors, and even malignant tumors, as cancer, may be successfully removed. Small cancers may sometimes be cured by repeated and long-continued freezing. Their growth may certainly be impeded by this means. Felons, if treated early in their course, may be cured by two or three freezings.

For freezing a felon, place the finger in a mixture of ice and salt, or surround it with cotton, saturate the cotton with ether or rhigoline, and blow it very strongly with a pair of bellows. This is a very good method when an apparatus for producing a fine spray is not at hand. The latter instrument facilitates the freezing very much if used with the bellows.

No harm results from repeated freezing if proper care is used in thawing the frozen parts. They should be kept immersed in cool water, or covered with cloths kept cool by frequent wetting with cold water, until the natural feeling is restored.

The application of ice is found extremely serviceable in many inflammatory diseases, and in some nervous affections. In inflammation of the brain, the ice cap is of inestimable value. Ice applied to the spine will check the convulsive spasms of chorea and hysteria when other remedies fail. In putrid sore throat, or malignant diphtheria, ice is a sovereign remedy. It should be applied to the neck externally, and held in small bits in the mouth. Small bits swallowed will sometimes relieve the pains of gastralgia.

Rubber bags are very convenient for applying ice or iced water; but their place can be very well supplied by dried bladders filled with pounded ice. The ice-cap is a double head-cap stuffed with pounded ice.

Some physicians recommend the application of ice to the spine in cases of congestive chill and paralysis, and in inflammation of the stomach, kidneys, uterus, and other internal organs. The real worth of such applications in these cases has yet to be determined by careful and repeated observations. We would not recommend an unskillful person to attempt to relieve a violent ague chill by rubbing ice on the patient's back, and we have some fears that a very skillful operator would hardly succeed to his entire satisfaction and that of the patient.

The snow bath, applied by rubbing the part vigorously with snow, is a useful application for restoring the circulation to frosted parts. In cases of extreme chilling or absolute freezing, there is perhaps no better remedy. Powdered ice may be used when snow cannot be readily procured.

MISCELLANEOUS BATHS, ETC.

VAPOR BATH.

This bath can be readily and successfully administered with such conveniences as every family possess. Place the patient in a cane-seat chair, having first taken the precaution to spread over the seat a dry towel. Surround the patient and the chair first with a woolen blanket, and then with two or three thick comfortables, drawing the blankets close around his neck, and allowing them to trail upon the floor so as to exclude the air as perfectly as possible. Now place under the chair a large pan or pail containing two or three quarts of boiling water. Let the blankets fall quickly so as to retain the rising vapor. After a minute or two, raise the blankets a little at one side and carefully place in the vessel a very hot brick or stone, dropping the blankets again as soon as possible to avoid the admission of cold air. Before the first brick or stone has cooled, add another, and so continue until the patient perspires freely. The amount of perspiration must be judged by the face and forehead, as much of the moisture on the skin beneath the blankets is condensed steam. Should the bath become at any time too hot, a little air may be admitted by raising the bottom of the blankets a little, being careful to avoid chilling the patient in so doing. The bath should seldom be continued more than half an hour, and fifteen to twenty minutes will usually accomplish all that is desired by the bath. If too long continued, it induces faintness. A too high temperature will be indicated by a strongly accelerated pulse, throbbing of the temples, flushed face, and headache. The head should be kept cool by a compress wet in cool water and often changed. The temperature of the bath should be from 100° to 115°. Unpleasant effects are sometimes produced at 120°.

After this bath, apply the tepid spray, rubbing wet-sheet, pail douche, or full bath. No time should be allowed to elapse after the blankets are removed before the concluding bath is applied, as the patient will chill. He should not be allowed to become chilly by exposure to cool air before the application of the spray, douche, or other bath, which should be followed by vigorous rubbing.

For "breaking up a cold," relieving rheumatism, soreness of the muscles from overexertion, and relaxing stiffened joints, this is a valuable agent. It may also be used to advantage in chronic diseases in which there is torpidity of the skin; but great care must be exercised to avoid excessive use, as too frequent repetitions of the bath produce debility.

This is a milder application than the hot-air bath, unless employed at a high temperature, 120° or more, when it becomes more severe.

In institutions where the bath is in daily requisition, a permanent arrangement for giving the bath is usually employed. It sometimes consists of a box in which the patient sits upon a stool, his head being allowed to remain outside by a suitable opening. A wet towel is placed around the neck to prevent the steam from rising about the head. Others prefer a box or small room large enough to admit the whole person, the whole body being subjected to the warm vapor. An opening guarded by a curtain is made in one side to allow the bather to inhale cool air if he should wish to do so, and to give the attendant access to the patient without chilling him by the admission of a large quantity of cold air. As in the simpler form of vapor bath, the head should be kept constantly cool by a cool wet compress often reapplied. Patients troubled with "rush of blood to the head," should be further protected by a large cool compress placed around the neck and the upper part of the chest.

Steam may be generated for these larger baths by boiling water in the box with a spirit-lamp or a gas-burner, or it may be conducted into the box by a rubber tube connected with a tight boiler.

RUSSIAN BATH.

This is essentially the same in effect as the vapor bath. It consists of a room filled with vapor, and so arranged that by transferring the patient from one point to another the heat may be gradually increased. It has no advantages not afforded by the simpler vapor bath. It is now much used in the larger cities. Probably as much harm as good results from the indiscriminate and reckless manner in which it is employed. Patients have been known to die in the bath of apoplexy induced by the excessive heat. It is followed by shampooing and cooling baths of various sorts.

HOT-AIR BATH.

In administering this bath, prepare the patient precisely as directed for the vapor bath. Instead of placing under the chair a vessel of hot water, place a large alcohol lamp or a small dish containing a few ounces of alcohol. When all is ready, light the lamp or alcohol, and carefully exclude the air. It is hardly necessary to suggest the propriety of putting the lamp in such a position as to insure safety from fire. If alcohol is used in an open dish, it is important to wipe the outside of the vessel quite free from any trace of the fluid, as otherwise it might be communicated to the floor or carpet. Also avoid spilling any portion in putting it in place, for the same reason. It is a very good precaution to place the dish containing the burning alcohol in a plate or shallow vessel containing a little water.

This bath should be conducted in the same manner as the vapor bath. A temperature of 140° to 160° is not at all disagreeable to the patient. At 170° or 180° the same effects are produced as in the vapor bath at 120°. The bath should be followed by cooling baths as directed for the vapor bath.

This is a very valuable remedy for the same class of diseases for which the vapor bath is recommended. It is of very great service in cases of dropsy, Bright's disease with poisoning from retained urea, and all cases in which a vigorous elimination by the skin is desired. It should not be continued longer than the vapor bath, and much harm may result from its too frequent employment. Like the vapor bath, this may be conducted in a suitable box with an opening for the head.

TURKISH BATH.

This is entirely analogous to the hot-air bath, though on a much more elaborate plan. The patient is gradually conducted from a temperature of 120° to that of 160° or even much more than 200°. The bath is concluded by shampooing, rubbing, cooling baths, and gradual cooling in a room maintained at a temperature of 70°.

The uses of this bath are the same as those of the hot-air bath. It has no advantages over it of very great importance, and is much more liable to produce injury by prolonged and frequent application. It generally occupies an hour, and by those who resort to it as a luxury, as did the ancient Romans, it is often prolonged to several hours.

The long-continued application of excessive heat to the body is a very unnatural process. It tends to produce permanent relaxation and debility of the cutaneous tissues, and the manner in which this bath is administered in Turkish bath establishments is productive of great harm. It is often presented to invalids as almost a panacea; and is given alike to the strong and vigorous, and the weak and debilitated.

The bath is certainly good in its place, but it is decidedly bad when abused. Many consider the hot-air bath greatly preferable since it obviates the necessity of inhaling superheated air, the effects of which upon the lungs are said to be injurious. The hot-air bath is doubtless safer.

ELECTRIC BATH.

Electricity may be more efficiently applied in connection with water than by itself. Water is a better conductor of electricity than the dry skin, and hence facilitates its communication to the body. The ordinary method of applying electricity is by attaching one pole of the battery to a metallic plate, placed in contact with some part of the body, while the circuit is completed by the application to the patient of a moist sponge connected with the other pole. The operator often holds one pole in his hand and applies the other hand, moistened, to the part to be treated. He is in this way enabled to judge very accurately of the strength of the current applied. The metallic plate is frequently placed at the feet of the patient, sometimes in a foot bath. The sponge may be applied to various parts of the body while the patient is in a sitz bath. For a general application of electricity the full bath is most convenient.

This bath is applicable to a very large variety of conditions. To describe them all would be to give nearly all the uses of electricity as a remedial agent, which does not come within the scope of this work. The electric full bath has been strongly recommended for the removal of mineral poisons from the body. Just how efficacious it is in this respect, we cannot confidently affirm. Probably its value has been somewhat exaggerated. Only the primary or galvanic current could be of any service in this direction.

Electricity is generally acknowledged to be a powerful remedial agent; but its use requires costly apparatus and much skill in application. It is necessary that the operator should not only understand the nature of diseases and the proper methods of applying electricity in treating them, but he must also thoroughly understand the general laws of electricity. The electric bath is as badly abused by quacks and charlatans as the Turkish bath. It should not be employed by unskillful persons; and for this and other reasons given, it is not well adapted to home use.

ELECTRO-VAPOR BATH.

This is a combination of the electric and the vapor bath, the electricity being applied to the body by means of the sponge, and metallic plates covered with moistened cloths. It is a valuable appliance if carefully used; but, like all effective modes of treatment, it is very liable to excessive use, which becomes abuse. It has been very highly lauded by certain specialists, and doubtless its' value has been unstintedly exaggerated. It is perhaps not well proven that its effects are greatly superior to the effects of the vapor bath and electric bath administered separately; and the latter mode would be more convenient, though consuming a little more time.

DRY RUBBING-SHEET.

Cover the patient with a soft, dry sheet in the same manner as directed for applying the wet sheet in the rubbing wet-sheet bath. Then rub lightly but briskly upon the outside of the sheet with the flat hand. Do not rub *with* the sheet, but over it. Continue the rubbing ten or fifteen minutes, going over the whole body several times, and not neglecting the arms, the hands, and the feet. This application may be administered daily with profit to nearly all patients. It should always follow any form of general bath in which water is employed, as a means of drying the body. It promotes activity of the skin, and equalizes the circulation.

DRY HAND-RUBBING.

This application is much the same in effect as the preceding, though a little more soothing, and hence better adapted to nervous patients. It consists in rubbing the body gently with the palm of the dry hand. The force of the rubbing should be nicely graduated to the condition of the patient. When employed to excite considerable activity of the skin, the rubbing may be accompanied with kneading of the abdomen, and light percussion of the surface.

Gentle rubbing of the skin is a very soothing process. It will frequently induce sleep when other means are ineffectual. Rubbing the back and limbs downward, and gentle rubbing of the temples, are very soothing to children and nervous invalids.

AIR BATH.

The air has a very soothing effect upon the body when allowed to come in contact with the entire surface. It answers a very valuable purpose when a water bath is impossible, or when the patient is too feeble to endure the application of water. A sleepless person will often fall into a sound and refreshing slumber after walking a few minutes in his room with the whole body exposed to the air. The effects of night labor upon literary people may be partially counteracted by the air bath. Benjamin Franklin was accustomed to pursue his writing to a late hour after divesting himself of his clothing, and he recommends the practice to others compelled to labor late with the pen.

SUN BATH.

The value of sunlight as a hygienic agent is so universally recognized—theoretically if not practically—that we need not devote space to its consideration in this connection. Sunlight is essential to the healthy performance of the vital functions, and must be equally important as an aid to remedial processes. This fact has been amply demonstrated by hospital experience, which shows a much larger percentage of recoveries in rooms abundantly exposed to the sun than in those secluded from its rays.

That the sun has a powerful influence upon the skin is shown by the great increase of pigment in that structure when freely exposed to the sunlight. This results from an increased activity of the.cutaneous tissues.

Experience has shown that the sun bath can be employed to advantage in most chronic diseases. The patient simply lies in a position in which the naked skin can be freely exposed to the rays of the sun. The head should be shaded. The bath should not be continued so long as to produce unpleasant effects either upon the skin or the general system. It may be accompanied and followed with the dry hand-rubbing.

SEA-BATHING.

Bathing in the sea is much practiced by fashionable people who make annual visits to the sea-coast for this purpose. It is no doubt useful, though many who participate in it would doubtless receive quite as much benefit if they took as many baths at home during the whole year as they take at the fashionable watering-places in a single week. It is a fine thing to be well washed once a year, however, if not more often.

As generally conducted, sea-bathing is not more beneficial than harmful. The dissipation accompanying it more than counterbalances what good might be gained. It is rather absurd to attribute any specific virtues to sea-water, as many do. Quite a large business is carried on in the evaporation of sea-water and the sale of the dirty residue, which is again dissolved in water and used in bathing by those who live too far inland to enjoy the benefits of bathing in the sea, or who prefer to take their sea-bath in their own private bath-room. Everything must have a counterfeit, and so this seasalt is imitated by base swindlers who prepare a mixture of chemicals just as powerful, but not quite so complicated, and less dirty, though certainly equally good. All of this trouble and swindling might be saved if people would only consider for a moment the fact that all the benefit they obtain from bathing is derived from the exercise, the temperature, and pure water, and not from any impurities which the water may chance to contain.

Sea-bathing is usually overdone. More benefit will be gained by one or two daily baths than by a half-dozen. Fifty baths in a single week are not equivalent to a single bath each in fifty weeks.

MEDICATED BATHS.

We have no faith in medicated baths in general. They are occasionally useful for the destruction of vermin, animal parasites, and perhaps in certain cases of skin disease. Generally, it is far better to take the limpid element "Simon pure," unadulterated. Many medicated baths have acquired great celebrity by the performance of cures really wonderful, but wholly attributable to water only, in spite of, rather than in conjunction with, the foreign medicament added.

OIL BATH.

Inunction was greatly practiced by the ancients in connection with the Roman and Turkish baths. It consists in rubbing the skin very thoroughly with some unctuous substance. Olive oil may be employed, but cosmoline or vaseline, two refined products of coal oil, are in some respects preferable. Olive oil cannot be obtained pure, except at almost fabulous prices. That sold in the drug stores as olive oil is really cotton-seed oil and mixtures of lard with various other vegetable oils.

A warm bath should first be administered. Then dry the patient, as usual, and apply the unguent, taking care to rub it in thoroughly. Simply greasing the surface is not the object sought. The skin and flesh should be worked, rubbed, and kneaded until the oil nearly disappears from the surface.

The object of this application is to supply the place of defective natural secretion of oleaginous material, to increase the activity of the skin, and to diminish susceptibility to cold. How this is accomplished, readily appears. The oil is a simple substitute for the sebaceous secretion, which is, in a certain class of diseases, notably deficient. The thorough manipulation of the skin which is necessary in applying the oil, and which is facilitated by a lubricant, directly promotes cutaneous activity. Whether the oil itself has any direct effect in increasing the functional activity of the skin cannot be positively affirmed, although it is reasonably supposable that the skin will act more nearly normal when a deficient element is supplied than when it is wanting. Oil is an excellent non-conductor; and invalids who are especially susceptible to cold may be rendered comfortable by the application of the oil bath.

The class of cases to which this remedy is applicable will be sufficiently well indicated by the purposes which the bath is supposed to subserve. It should not be used indiscriminately. Once or twice a week is sufficiently often to make the application, and each should be followed by a warm bath with fine soap, two or three days after.

NOVEL BATHS.

Numerous substances have been employed in bathing, under the idea that they possessed peculiar specific virtues; the following are some of the chief:—

Mud Bath.—Immersion of the body in warm mud has been a favorite practice at several places in Italy, France, Germany, and other countries. The effects are not very different from those of any warm bath, and are said to be very pleasant, by those who have taken them. If the mud were not medicated, this kind of bath would not be especially objectionable for those who could enjoy it.

Earth Bath.—Burying the body in the moist earth has also been practiced. We have known of one instance in which this remedy was successfully used in the treatment of ague.

Bees' eggs, milk, blood, wine, sand, and *gelatine* have also been employed by different nations, at different periods, in bathing. None of these applications are superior to pure water, which all nature recognizes as the proper material for bathing purposes.

ENEMA.

Fecal accumulations in the lower bowel are more quickly and easily removed by an enema of warm water than by any purgative, laxative, or cathartic ever discovered or invented; and the use of this remedy is never accompanied by the unpleasant and painful griping and tenesmus which often accompany the use of cathartics. The administration is a trifle more troublesome, but the results are enough superior to more than repay the inconvenience. The fountain syringe is far preferable to any other for administering injections. Water about blood-warm should be used when the purpose is to relieve constipation, and a considerable quantity—one to three pints, or more—may be used. The water should be retained for a few minutes, while the bowels are kneaded and shaken. In hemorrhage and inflammation of the lower bowel, cool or cold clysters should be employed, and should be retained as long as possible. The copious cool enema is a valuable antiphlogistic remedy used in conjunction with the cool bath in cases of violent febrile excitement, as typhoid fever, when the temperature rises above 103° F.

The enema is a most perfect substitute for purgatives in general. Cases are very rare in which a cathartic drug will be found necessary if the enema is properly used. But the enema may become a source of mischief if abused. If habitually relied upon to secure a movement of the bowels for a long time, the bowels lose their activity, and the most obstinate constipation sometimes results, precisely as from the prolonged use of purgatives.

WATER EMETIC.

Warm water at about 92°—not hot water—is a most excellent emetic if taken in sufficient quantity. It is prompt in action, and is unaccompanied by the painful nausea, retching, and straining produced by most other emetics. From half a pint to one or two quarts is required to produce emesis. The patient should slowly swallow a tumblerful, then rest two or three minutes, and swallow another, so continuing to drink for ten minutes or more. As soon as the slightest disposition to vomit is felt—or even if it is not felt, after a considerable quantity of water has been taken—the patient should touch the back part of his mouth with the end of his finger or a feather, as far down as he can reach. This will usually excite the desired action. If it does not, all that need be done is to continue drinking. A little salt added to the water will make it more sickening, and will do no particular harm, as it is thrown out again.

It is not claimed that the warm-water emetic can replace all other emetics in *all cases*. When instant vomiting is necessary, as in cases of poisoning, some more prompt emetic may be used with it. But for all ordinary purposes, it clearly has no rival.

DRY HOT APPLICATIONS.

The use of fomentations is often less convenient or desirable than dry applications of heat, which may be made in a variety of ways. Bottles, jugs, or rubber bags, filled with hot water, hot bricks or stones, wrapped in papers or cloths, hot cloths, bags filled with hot sand, salt, or corn meal, are all convenient methods of applying dry heat.

A few suggestions with reference to the manner of using hot applications may be useful. In applying heat to the feet when the circulation in those organs is defective, it is frequently insufficient to apply the heat to the bottoms of the feet, only. For this reason, jugs or bottles and stones are often applied without effecting any satisfactory results. A much more efficient method is the following: Heat to a suitable temperature two or three pounds of corn meal or salt. Place the salt or meal in a bag sufficiently large to envelop the feet. After distributing it evenly through the bag, wrap the latter about the feet and cover them with a woolen blanket. A rubber bag partially filled with hot water is an excellent appliance for use in cases of neuralgia, toothache, and nearly all acute pains in the region of the head, as it will conform so perfectly to the shape of the part to which it is applied, and may be used as a pillow.

As a general rule, hot applications should not be continued more than an hour or two, at longest, without, at least, a transient application of a lower temperature. Too prolonged an application may result in injury to the part.

WATER-DRINKING.

As a remedial agent, water is of far greater value than any other liquid taken into the stomach. Its uses in preserving health have been previously noticed. Under ordinary circumstances, a person in health who discards irritating condiments from his diet seldom requires drink. Many persons take no drink whatever during the winter months. But drinking is healthful, and pure water of proper temperature may be taken by any one in health or disease if it is taken in the proper manner. Drinking at meals is an unwholesome practice. Drinking large quantities of iced water is unhealthful. Cold water should not be taken freely when the drinker is hot or exhausted. The thirst will be quenched as readily by slowly sipping a small quantity. In fevers, water should be freely allowed. A glass of cool water taken half an hour before breakfast is an excellent remedy for habitual constipation.

Water-drinking may be made a means of bathing the internal structures, as external applications bathe the outside. Water is rapidly absorbed by the mucous membrane of the stomach, and, passing through the circulation, it dissolves many impurities, and is eliminated chiefly by the kidneys and skin. It can be used with benefit in connection with the vapor bath, hot-air bath, and all baths in which sweating is induced. It should not be used in such great excess as it was employed by the early hydropathists, however, whose patients drank from ten to thirty glasses of water a day.

Free drinking of water is useful in cases in which the urine is scanty and irritating. It gives relief by diluting the urinary excretions.

HOW TO MAKE A FILTER.

For drinking, and for all ordinary purposes, it is of the greatest importance that water should be as pure as possible. When water which is nearly soft, and wholly free from organic impurities, cannot be obtained from wells or springs, filtered rain water should be employed. A very useful filter can be easily and cheaply constructed in the following manner :—

Make a hole low down in the side, or in the bottom, of a large earthen jar or flower-pot. Place in the bottom of the vessel a few clean stones about the size of eggs. Fill the jar to within two or three inches of the top with equal parts of fine, clean gravel and pulverized charcoal. Cover the jar with a clean, white cloth, securing the edges by a string drawn about the top. The center of the cloth cover should be allowed to hang down into the vessel so as to form a hollow into which the water may be poured, the cloth serving as a strainer to remove the coarser dirt. The cloth should be frequently cleansed, and the gravel and charcoal should be renewed at least once a year.

We invite you to view the complete
selection of titles we publish at:

www.LNFBooks.com

or write or email us your praises,
reactions, or thoughts about this
or any other book we publish at:

TEACH Services, Inc.
P.O. Box 954
Ringgold, GA 30736

info@TEACHServices.com

CPSIA information can be obtained at www.ICGtesting.com
Printed in the USA
LVOW100944260113

317271LV00001B/26/P